INTRODUCTION

There has never been a better ti to be diagnosed with either Type 1 or Type 2 diabete   iis fact while watching *Coronation*   ɘrt during the commercials showed   ɳg machine, now available to buy (ve moved on from the way things used to be. Even forty years ago there wasn't the knowledge that high glucose levels cause other health problems. I wish there had of been, as now I'm living with the consequences of years of poor diabetes control in the form of eye and nerve problems. I'll say it again – we are so lucky to be able to use available knowledge and technology to prevent or delay complications of diabetes in this day and age!

When I was first diagnosed with Type 1 diabetes aged 10, I had no idea what it was or what it meant for the future, so I didn't really care about looking after it. I did my two injections of insulin per day using a glass syringe and stainless steel needle (that had to be sharpened on a pumice stone and sterilised in surgical spirit), and I did a urine test for glucose morning and evening – that was that. If the urine test turned orange, I knew I was in trouble, but there was no advice about reducing a high blood sugar (glucose) level. I saw a diabetes specialist once a year who said my condition was incredibly difficult to control, and I was advised that if I did any sport at school I needed to eat a chocolate bar beforehand. That was the sum total of the diabetes care I received forty years ago.

There is a phrase, 'Laughter is the best medicine.' Well, it is, but I'd rank insulin (the hormone that controls *blood glucose* levels) or Metformin (prescribed for Type 2 diabetes) right up there too. 'So, having available treatments is brilliant,' I hear you cry. It certainly is and I, for one, wouldn't be here without them. But there is unfortunately a cruel irony; a bitter-sweet twist: by staying alive longer with available treatments for diabetes, the ravages of long-term higher than normal blood glucose (BG) levels take their toll in the form of complications.

Believe me, this is not one of those 'slap on the wrist' warnings that you should look after yourself, or else, without explaining why or how. I know from personal experience that this sort of finger-wagging approach to manging diabetes can send a person running and screaming in the opposite direction. (This is how those who must be obeyed used to do it in the 1970s and I was often 'told off'). What I hope to do is explain what diabetes is, and why and how it CAN be managed to prevent or significantly delay the development of any complications. The ultimate goal for me is to provide you with insight, experience and information so you can lead a happy, healthy life with diabetes.

So, what *is* diabetes?

Diabetes is a change in your body chemistry which causes there to be too much glucose in the blood. This is because of a lack of the hormone, insulin, or because insulin can't work properly in the body. There are two kinds of diabetes. Type 1 happens when the body attacks its own insulin-producing cells in the pancreas (an organ in the abdomen) so that little or no insulin is made – this is a permanent situation (thought to be triggered by a virus) known as *auto-immune* destruction so Type 1 diabetes can't be cured. Type 2 diabetes is a complex condition involving a number of factors as well as high blood glucose levels, usually triggered by body weight and a lack of physical activity. With this condition there is usually a

DIABETES?
KEEP CALM AND
TAKE CONTROL

by Dr Val Wilson

For Neil

CONTENTS

Introduction	1–9
Living with diabetes	10–27
A rollercoaster of emotions	28–59
How will diabetes affect me?	60–115
Getting back control	116–159
Diet and exercise	160–171
Reversing Type 2 diabetes	172–188
What diabetes care should I receive?	189–199
Young and old	200–229
Helpful hints, recipes and tips	230–231
Recipes	232–267
Useful contacts	268–272
Notes	273–275
Further reading	276–278
Glossary of terms	279–294
Index	295–307

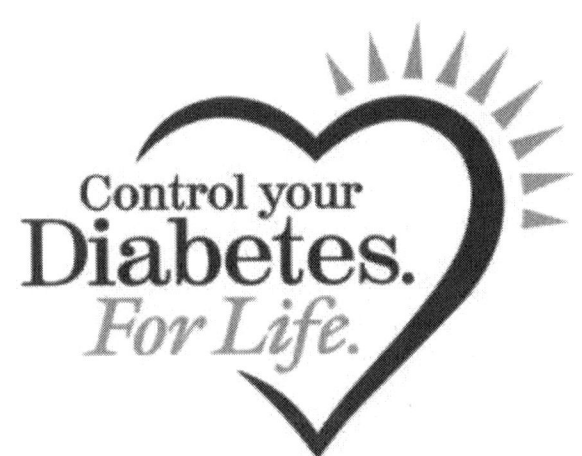

Control your
Diabetes.
For Life.

combined alteration in the amount of insulin produced when blood glucose levels are too high and a reduced response to insulin in the body cells so that it can't do its job properly.

Although the medical profession may beg to differ, I've always believed that the best person to educate others about diabetes is someone who actually has the condition because 'you don't get it 'till you get it'. This does, of course, depend on the teacher and their own understanding of the condition: In 1850, for example, a diabetes consultant advised his patients that they needed to eat vast quantities of sugar to replace what was being lost in their urine! The irony was, he was also diabetic and his own treatment killed him and most of his patients.

If you are wondering what makes me such an expert – you already know that I have diabetes – I've also studied for a couple of qualifications in diabetes health education. Initially I did this with the intention of helping myself rather than other people, but I soon found my knowledge was useful in this respect. Here's one example:

> A friend told me that her husband, Dave, had recently been diagnosed with Type 2 diabetes. Dave was tired, thirsty, taking frequent trips to the toilet to empty his bladder, and began experiencing blurred vision and numbness in his feet and lower legs. He'd ignored these symptoms for several months, putting them down to just getting older. During a routine visit to the dentist, Dave was advised to go and see his GP because high glucose levels had led to thrush (a yeast infection) in his mouth. A few weeks later Dave was finally diagnosed with Type 2 diabetes and began taking Metformin tablets to lower his BG levels. He felt better almost immediately but because he felt better, Dave thought his diabetes had gone away. One day Dave's wife told me, 'He's so much better now, but he feels ill if he eats a few doughnuts.' Sadly, no one had told Dave about avoiding sweet foods unless he had the symptoms of low BG such as

dizziness, sweating, shaking, and confusion. I explained that taking Metformin does not mean that Type 2 diabetes goes away, or that by taking a tablet, sweet foods can be eaten like before Dave had diabetes. Dave said he hadn't known what or who to ask and his doctors and nurse were busy, with little time to make things clear.

Needing to visit the bathroom more often and having a raging thirst are major symptoms of diabetes, although this can be much less obvious in Type 2 diabetes and can last for years, compared with the dramatic thirst and urination seen in Type 1. In the 17th century diabetes was described as 'the pissing evil' (remembering that there was no treatment at the time). This sums up perfectly the constant flow of urine when there is too much glucose present before diabetes is diagnosed. The thirst and need to urinate happens because the body is trying to flush all the glucose (that it can't use without the help of insulin) out the body. Without insulin or glucose-lowering tablets, glucose (sugar) can't be used by the body for energy.

Unfortunately, there's no way to make medical matters exciting. As I've mentioned, there are two main types of diabetes that happen for different reasons, but both ultimately lead to increased blood glucose (BG) levels if left untreated. Type 1 diabetes is very quick to develop and, if BG levels become dangerously high, may lead to a medical emergency. Type 2 diabetes may take up to twelve years to develop fully, but because the level of glucose in the blood is higher than normal, complications such as heart disease may occur during that time. Imagine the heart trying to pump thick syrup around the body and you can see why trying to keep BG levels under control is so important: high blood glucose levels thicken the blood and make it sticky.

So, to recap, there are two main types of diabetes. *Type 1 diabetes* happens when the body no longer produces the hormone insulin to control BG levels because the insulin-producing part of the pancreas is attacked by the body's own defence mechanisms (*auto-immune attack*). This attack continues throughout the person's life meaning that this condition is not reversible. This used to be called 'child onset diabetes' because it mainly happens in young people.

The second kind is *Type 2 diabetes*. Type 2 is a different form of the condition with its own causes and effects. It is a complex disorder resulting in insulin (a hormone produced by the pancreas) not being able to be used correctly by the body to bring BG levels under control. This used to be seen most often in people over forty years of age, especially the elderly where the pancreas had begun to wear out.

Today Type 2 diabetes is recognised as a condition related to lifestyle as it is now often seen in people who are overweight and inactive (even children), resulting in more and more insulin being produced to bring BG levels down. This imbalance can be reversed in many cases with lifestyle change. It is a very sad fact that for these reasons, Type 2 diabetes in children is steadily increasing.

There is also a form of diabetes that develops from the twentieth week of pregnancy because hormonal changes block the normal action of insulin, but this condition (*gestational diabetes*) disappears after the birth. However, this does increase the risk of developing Type 2 diabetes within 15 years of the pregnancy in over half of women who have had gestational diabetes. A rare condition called *diabetes insipidus* has similar symptoms of increased thirst and frequent urination but when tested, the blood and urine do not contain an abnormal amount of glucose.

To sum up, diabetes occurs when there is a change in the way the body can use glucose, causing there to be too much glucose in the blood and a lack of insulin to correct this imbalance.

How many people have diabetes?

Don't worry – you are not alone and you don't have to suffer in silence. Around 700 people a day are diagnosed with diabetes – that's the equivalent of one every two minutes. In January, 2016 Diabetes UK announced that 4 million people now have diabetes of one form or another in the UK. Globally this figure is currently 415 million, although this does not include children with the condition.

Because Type 2 diabetes is usually related to lifestyle and people are living longer now with serious medical conditions that can be managed, this accounts for 90 percent of cases. The remaining 10 percent have Type 1 diabetes, but this is now also on the increase.

Although the statistics don't include them, there are an estimated 31,500 children and young people with diabetes in the UK, meaning around 2 in every 1,000 children have diabetes (the majority with Type 1). This estimate has been made based on the number attending diabetes clinics especially for young people, but this figure could be as high as 42,000 as some 15–19 year-olds attend an adult diabetes clinic. Around 95% of these children and young adults have Type 1 and the remainder have Type 2 diabetes. In the year 2000, the first cases of Type 2 diabetes were diagnosed in overweight female children as young as 7 years old. There are slightly more boys than girls with Type 1, but more girls than boys develop Type 2.

FACT: GP surgeries now offer annual health checks where you can take a urine sample to be tested for glucose, even if you haven't had any symptoms of diabetes.

Type 2 diabetes in the UK is often managed by you and your GP rather than having appointments with a diabetes consultant at a hospital. This is called PRIMARY CARE. This is to make sure you are looked after by health professionals who can help you keep good control of your BG, blood pressure and cholesterol to reduce the risk of developing complications of diabetes.

Getting your diabetes care from your GP and Practice Nurse has the main advantages for you of being able to phone for an appointment whenever you need it rather than just seeing a consultant every six months or yearly. Your GP surgery also has easy access to your medical notes and history and they know you better than a much more impersonal hospital clinic where you may not see the same health professional each time you have an appointment. This also has the disadvantage of having to explain details about yourself and your diabetes, and if you have to attend several clinics, this can be tiresome because your medical notes are not shared between hospitals.

FACT: You may think that Type 2 diabetes is not as serious as Type 1 diabetes. This is not the case. Having Type 2 diabetes increases the risk of developing heart disease, so having good control of BG, blood pressure and cholesterol levels is very important.

How many people don't know they have diabetes?

I apologise for all these facts and figures, but they are a good way of showing how many people are affected by diabetes. Because Type 2 diabetes is developing so often in what is known as 'Western society' – where people eat a high calorie, high-fat diet and do little or no exercise, diabetes has reached epidemic proportions worldwide. The symptoms are mild and are often ignored for years before Type 2 diabetes is diagnosed.

Experts think that one person in every 16 now has Type 2 diabetes without knowing it. Like Dave, who I mentioned earlier, the symptoms may be put down to getting older or being tired because of work or life stresses. The trouble with having high BG levels over many months, or even years, is that this can eventually cause damage to blood vessels and nerves – and there are blood vessels and nerves all over the body, so any part of you can be affected by diabetes. This means it's important to go to your doctor with any symptoms – like an increased thirst or frequent visits to the toilet – so that diabetes can be diagnosed as soon as possible.

About this book

This book has been written to help you understand your diagnosis so you can manage and live with your diabetes as well as possible. The things that you need to know are covered in each chapter with important words in italics because they also appear in the glossary at the end of the book with more explanation. I have included loads of facts and tips that appear in bold throughout, and there's an extensive index that you will hopefully find useful. Case studies are also used frequently to show experiences of diabetes-related issues you might be dealing with.

I can honestly say that you never stop learning when you have diabetes and it's not always simple. Following diagnosis and the start of appropriate treatment there is blood glucose (BG) monitoring, medication, diet and exercise to get to grips with – a complete lifestyle change. *Diabetes? Keep Calm and Take Control* gives you answers to making these changes so you can be in control of your diabetes rather than it being in control of you.

LIVING WITH DIABETES

'The worse thing for me was being told that I'd have diabetes for the rest of my life.'

So, you have diabetes? You are probably feeling depressed and angry, thinking, 'Why me?' This is a perfectly normal reaction. What is different in your case is that you've made the first positive step to taking control by buying this book. The way you deal with your diabetes is very personal and it's never too late to start having a better understanding of how it affects you – knowledge is your greatest weapon. This can be the difference between diabetes becoming a big tiresome deal in your life or a condition that you are confident you can manage and control well.

Symptoms

You may wonder why I'm mentioning the symptoms of diabetes when you've already been through this bit, had your diagnosis and you're now taking medication. The reason this section is here is because diabetes does far less damage to the body if it can be diagnosed early. By knowing the symptoms, which can be different for other people to those you experienced, you might be able to advise someone else to see their doctor sooner rather than later.

Case Study

Paula Brown noticed that her 10 year-old daughter, Natalie, seemed to be drinking more and was very tired all the time. Paula was worried that Natalie had also lost a lot of weight very quickly, although she had actually been eating more, saying she was hungry. After a few weeks Natalie began to wet the bed, even though she was emptying her bladder at bedtime. Paula mentioned these symptoms to the family GP, but he reassured her that it was probably only a urine or bladder infection and that Natalie should be given plenty of fluids. After a fortnight Natalie's symptoms seemed worse and Paula took her to see a different GP in the practice. He did a urine test and told Paula that it contained a high amount of glucose. Natalie was admitted to hospital, diagnosed with Type 1 diabetes, and insulin injections were started to bring her glucose (sugar) levels under control. After seeing the hospital diabetes nurse, Natalie began to manage her Type 1 diabetes very successfully at home and at school.

Case Study

John Taylor was 55, rather overweight and took little exercise as a security guard who sat watching CCTV footage for most of the day. He was feeling itchy much of the time and his wife, Maureen, thought he might be having a reaction to their washing powder, so she changed it. Four months passed and John was now feeling he had no energy, despite drinking a bottle of Lucozade every day – liquid glucose. As the time went on, John convinced himself he felt under the weather because of the stresses and strains of his job. John hated going to the doctor because she always commented on his weight, so he forced himself to carry on. One weekend about a year after John first complained of constant itching, he was mowing the small front lawn when he collapsed. Maureen called an ambulance and, after tests at the hospital, John was told he had Type 2 diabetes. Maureen wished she'd encouraged John to see his doctor about the itching.

As you can see, Natalie and John both had very different symptoms. Type 1 diabetes tends to make itself known within weeks or months, whereas Type 2 diabetes (according to Diabetes UK) can take up to 12 years before it is finally diagnosed as the symptoms can be subtle and are often ignored.

The main symptoms that you may be familiar with are feeling very thirsty and needing to wee far more frequently than usual. This happens because your body cannot deal with sugar (glucose) when insulin is not produced in Type 1 diabetes, or because insulin cannot be used properly by the body in Type 2 diabetes. When insulin isn't available in this way, glucose levels build up in the blood and this spills over into the urine, causing us to drink more and more to replace the fluids and flush the glucose out. This can only be treated by replacing the missing insulin by injection or taking glucose-lowering medications.

WHAT ARE THE MAIN SYMPTOMS OF DIABETES?

You may have experienced all or only some of these before your diagnosis:

- Increased thirst.
- Passing large quantities of urine, especially at night.
- Dehydration (through loss of fluids).
- Tiredness and lethargy.
- Blurred vision.
- General itching and an increase in episodes of thrush (a yeast infection).
- Weight loss.

Why glucose is the issue

Your body uses glucose for energy to power your brain, muscles and chemical reactions. *Glucose* is a type of sugar that comes from the breakdown of carbohydrates like bread, potatoes and pasta. *Sugar* is a simple carbohydrate that breaks down into glucose in the body. Eating either glucose or sugar – or the carbohydrates they become as they are processed by the body – increases blood glucose (BG) levels.

The hormone insulin is released into the bloodstream by the pancreas (an organ in the abdomen) to control the level of glucose. See insulin as the burly doorman that allows glucose to enter into muscle or fat cells. Without insulin, the cells have no available fuel, although there is plenty of glucose waiting to be let in. This starvation of the cells is why there is such rapid weight loss in people with Type 1 diabetes before diagnosis – because BG levels are extremely high and there is little or no insulin being produced. With Type 2 diabetes where there is obesity, the fat around body cells stops insulin working correctly, so more and more insulin is produced. Insulin is therefore very necessary – we cannot do without it and it has many important jobs in the body.

FACT: As well as controlling BG levels, insulin also supports the formation of fat and muscle; it enables the storage of glucose in the liver as *glycogen* for later use; and it prevents protein (needed for cell growth) from being broken down.

Having diabetes means your body can no longer deal with glucose in the same way because there is either a lack of insulin to keep glucose within normal limits (Type 1 diabetes), or because the insulin produced cannot work properly (Type 2 diabetes).

When your doctor tells you that you have diabetes this is because tests have shown excessive glucose levels in your blood due to inadequate available insulin. Glucose in the blood is measured in millimoles per litre (mmol/L). I talk about your own BG tests to self-manage diabetes later, but in terms of diagnosis, any ONE of the following results is used by doctors to decide whether someone has diabetes or not:

- When the glucose level of a blood *plasma* sample (the liquid part of blood) is <u>11 mmol/L</u> or higher.
- When there is a BG measurement of 6.1 mmol/L after the person has <u>fasted</u> for 10 hours and drunk only water.
- When a glucose tolerance test shows a plasma glucose level higher than <u>11 mmol/L</u> two hours after drinking 75 grams of glucose dissolved in water.
- If BG levels are high but there are NO SYMPTOMS of diabetes, such as increased thirst and a need to urinate more often, a second test is necessary to confirm a diagnosis of diabetes.

Diagnosis – Why me?

To answer the question, 'Why me?' we have to go into matters like already having associated medical conditions, genetic factors and lifestyle issues that make a person more likely to develop diabetes. Medical conditions (such certain cancers) where part of the pancreas is removed means diabetes develops, but it is less severe because the hormone called *glycogen* (which raises BG levels in the body) is also reduced, meaning you can function with less insulin.

Other *auto-immune* conditions (where the body's immune system attacks healthy tissue) are often also diagnosed before or after Type 1 diabetes (an auto-immune disease). These include under- and over-active thyroid conditions, asthma, *coeliac disease* (an intolerance to gluten in wheat), and *psoriasis* (a condition affecting the skin and joints).

Diabetes is more likely to develop in people with certain genetic factors. Having a parent with Type 1 diabetes increases the odds of also developing diabetes by 3–4%. If you have an identical twin with Type 1 you have a 20% chance of also getting the condition, but this drops to 5% if you are one of non-identical twins. If your brothers and sisters are different ages to you (i.e., not identical or twins) you have a less than 1% chance of developing Type 1 diabetes.

In terms of Type 2 diabetes, having an identical twin with the condition means you have a 90% chance of also developing it. If one of your parents has Type 2 you are 40% more likely to also develop the condition in your lifetime and if both your parents have Type 2 this likelihood rises to 50%.

Racial and ethnic minorities – defined as American Indians and Alaska Americans; Black or African Americans; Hispanics or Latins; and Asian Americans are MORE LIKELY to develop diabetes than Whites and some minority groups. Figures show that Type 2 diabetes develops more often in the Asian population, with 16% of Asians in the UK affected.

Medical conditions causing increased levels of other hormones can have a significant effect on the way insulin works, meaning the body has to produce more insulin to make BG levels normal (*glucose intolerance*) and diabetes may develop due to genetic factors. If you are prescribed anti-inflammatory medicines such as *hydro-cortisone* or *prednisone* for conditions such as severe asthma, arthritis, or inflammatory bowel disease, this could increase your chances of developing diabetes.

Certain drugs can also have the side effect of increasing BG levels. These include some blood pressure medications (especially *bendrofluozide*) and the water tablets, *thiazide*, raise BG levels and can lead to diabetes if you are genetically susceptible to developing the condition.

Lifestyle factors such as being overweight and having a high Body Mass Index (BMI), as well as doing little or no exercise mean you are much more likely to develop Type 2 diabetes than if you maintain a healthy weight and are physically active. We know this because people who live in countries who don't traditionally eat fast food or junk food, and who are very active tend to have a much lower risk of developing Type 2 diabetes.

A population that actually went from eating fish and vegetables to eating higher fat, higher calorie foods when they became rich due to mineral deposits in their land then went on to have a much higher number of people who developed Type 2 diabetes. This means that changing your lifestyle from eating healthy foods and being active to eating convenience foods and junk foods that tend to be high in calories and fat can, over time and in combination with little or no exercise, make you much more likely to develop Type 2 diabetes at some time in your life.

Your Body Mass Index (or BMI) is a measurement that uses your height and weight to work out if you're healthy although this can be a problem for people with a large amount of muscle – like rugby players, as muscle weighs heavier than fat. A person with a BMI of 20–24.9 is considered to be of normal weight whereas a BMI of 25–29.9 is classed as overweight. A BMI of 30 and above is considered obese.

Your BMI can be calculated by dividing your weight in kilograms by the square of your height in metres, so if you are a man who is 6 feet tall (1.83 metres) weighing 14 stone 2 pounds (90 kilograms), your BMI is 27.

Studies have shown that people with a BMI of 35 and above are 100 times more likely to develop Type 2 diabetes than people with a BMI of 22 or less. The length of time that a person is obese is also important: the longer they are obese the more likely they are to develop Type 2 diabetes.

FACT: Being overweight means insulin can't work properly in the cells of the body. This is called *insulin resistance.*

FACT: If you are a woman with a waist measurement of over 35 inches or a man whose waist measures over 40 inches, you are at increased risk of developing Type 2 diabetes and heart disease.

As I've previously mentioned, having a sedentary lifestyle (meaning taking little or no exercise) significantly increases the chance of developing Type 2 diabetes, especially in association with obesity. Even if someone is slim, Type 2 can still occur if they take little or no exercise. Studies show that a Type 2 diagnosis happens far more often in people who do not exercise than in those who are fairly active.

A key factor indicating an increased risk of developing Type 2 diabetes is the excess body fat that sits around the waistline, making the person appear apple-shaped rather than pear-shaped. Insulin cannot work properly when there is a lot of fat present around the body cells and excess fat in the mid-section of the body has the greatest effect on the working ability of insulin to reduce BG levels.

The good news is that fat around the waistline area of the body (known as *visceral fat*) is much easier to lose when you diet than fat elsewhere in the body. This is because when you reduce your calorie intake and become more physically active, the fat stored in this area is the first to be used. Make sure you consult your doctor if you're planning to start dieting and before beginning a new exercise regime.

Case Study

Joan Ralph was 44 and worked in an office. She had put on weight recently after eating takeaway meals most nights instead of cooking and she was too tired to do very much in the way of exercise. Joan told herself that she wasn't actually overweight, just a few pounds heavier. One day Joan went to the supermarket and saw that Diabetes UK had a stall outside. After talking to them she found she was at increased risk of developing Type 2 diabetes because her mother had the condition. This was the wake-up call Joan needed to start eating more healthily and begin using an exercise bike in front of the television for twenty minutes every evening. This helped her lose the weight she had gained, plus a bit extra. Joan found she actually enjoyed the exercise as she felt much better, so she made this part of her lifestyle.

Case Study

Ruth Fairfax had always considered herself healthy. When she was 28 she had her first baby and developed difficult to manage gestational diabetes – she was told that her baby would be large because of her increased BG levels. When Ruth's baby, Sarah, was born she weighed 12 pounds. When Sarah was 18 she developed Type 1 diabetes. She already had an over-active thyroid gland and Sarah's consultant told her that both conditions were due to her own immune system attacking healthy tissue in her body. Her mother, Ruth, had developed Type 2 diabetes 13 years after having Sarah because of her gestational diabetes, which put her at an increased risk of having the condition. Ruth's parents also developed Type 2 diabetes within a year of one another because they were elderly and much less active. Ruth was shocked to realise that three generations of her family had diabetes due to different causes.

FACT: Obese men are at higher risk of developing Type 2 diabetes and dangerous levels of liver fats than women.

Your local government health website helps you assess your risk of developing Type 2 diabetes in two minutes by entering your height, weight and waistline measurement. You can also find out about healthy eating and how to fit more physical activity into your lifestyle. Because the advice is the same across all areas of the country, and in case you can't find this information, the web address for my local area which you can use to access this information is:

medway.gov.uk/diabetes

Common myths and misconceptions

There are lots of myths about diabetes and many misunderstandings. I once found a website on the Internet set up for parents of children with Type 1 diabetes. I won't say what it was called, but it stated that this condition is caused by children eating too many sweets. I was shocked and annoyed, so I contacted them and politely suggested that this information was wrong, giving the real cause – auto-immune destruction of the insulin-producing cells of the pancreas triggered, scientists currently agree, by a virus. This virus prevents the survival of any new insulin-producing cells that form for the rest of the person's life.

I am pleased to say that after I contacted the person who had put this false information out there blaming parents for giving their children sweets and making them ill, the website promptly disappeared from the Internet. This is obviously a case of misinformation, but unfortunately there's a lot of it about, perhaps because over time ideas change, new understandings form, and science shows the truth from the fiction. Here are some more myths I'm keen to bust

DIABETES IS CAUSED BY STRESS

Stress may be a trigger for diabetes to start because the insulin-producing cells of the pancreas (the *islet cells*) are already failing to produce enough insulin hormone for the body's needs, making someone more likely to develop the condition. The hormones released when you are stressed once you have diabetes cause your BG to go up by increasing the amount of glucose that's available to the muscles.

Stress is a situation where you need energy and, if you can work it off, it's a good thing. But when you are stressed in combination with diabetes (say, if you've had an argument with someone), your body can't deal with this excess glucose you don't use. If you are stressed over a longer period and it's not just a one-off, it is a good idea to check your BG more often as you may need to increase your insulin, or speak to your diabetes nurse if you have Type 2 diabetes (and are not prescribed insulin) so she can adjust your medication.

HAVING DIABETES MEANS YOU CAN'T EAT SWEET THINGS

There are times, such as when your BG is low, that you NEED to eat something sweet in order to bring your BG back up to a normal level. This does not mean that eating sweets to avoid hypoglycaemia (low BG levels) should be used as an excuse to family and friends (I've known several people who keep sweets in their desks at work for 'emergencies' but dip into them all day long).

If you have Type 2 diabetes and take tablets, or use diet and exercise to lower your BG, you have less opportunity for eating sweet things for pleasure rather than necessity because you don't have the same opportunity to bring your glucose down again in the way that people who take insulin do.

Current thinking in Type 1 diabetes suggests that insulin dosages should be given for the carbohydrate content of the food you eat. This is known as Dosage Adjustment For Normal Eating, or DAFNE for short. I will go into this in more detail later but the good news is that, if you eat a couple of biscuits at, for example, 50 grams of carbohydrate, as long as you give yourself the right amount of insulin to cover the carbohydrate you eat, you can eat normally without restrictions (once you've been on the DAFNE course for managing Type 1 diabetes).

EVERY TIME YOU HAVE A HYPO SOME BRAIN CELLS DIE OFF

Hypoglycaemia (low BG levels) is a lack of glucose to fuel the brain and muscles so, unsurprisingly, you can feel tired, shaky, and very confused, often with a major lasting headache. Mild to moderate hypos, where you can eat or drink something sweet to bring yourself out of it, are NOT harmful to the brain.

Severe hypos, resulting in becoming unconscious and in some case, having an epileptic-like fit, require the assistance of another person in the form of giving an injection of *Glucagen*. This is the same as the glucose stored in the liver and it works very quickly to increase BG, bringing the individual out of unconsciousness but feeling very delicate. Brain scans following these very severe events have shown some loss of grey matter (brain cells). However, the brain is very good at compensating for any loss and rapidly develops new connections so any effect on mental function is minimal.

YOU CAN ACHIEVE PERFECT CONTROL OF BLOOD GLUCOSE LEVELS

Control is a word you'll hear many times in connection with your diabetes – it's even in the title of this book! There is no such thing as perfect control – if you had it you wouldn't have diabetes because your body would be able to keep BG levels within normal limits on its own. Health professionals (your GP, Practice Nurse, diabetes consultant and diabetes nurse) like you to aim for NORMAL to GOOD control, although this is not always easy if you have repeated infections and/or depression or *brittle diabetes* (diabetes that is very difficult to control) that increases your BG levels.

Normal to good control means achieving BG readings of between 5.0–8.3 mmol/L so the amount of glucose that sticks to your red blood cells over a three-month period (your *HbA1c* or *haemoglobin A1c* measurement) is between 5–7% (31–53 mmol/L). Fair control is a result between 7–8% (53–64 mmol/L) and poor control is a result of 9% (75 mmol/L) and upwards. In the United States your HbA1c is known as the eAG (or average blood glucose) and this is expressed as a percentage. However, HbA1c measurement does not record any highs and lows as in your day to day blood tests for diabetes management. A result in the good range is highly motivating and proves that you are doing a great job.

FACT: The occasional high or low BG level is to be expected so don't let it throw you. Continue to manage your diabetes as you have been taught and you will be taking control of your condition.

HAVING TO TAKE INSULIN FOR TYPE 2 DIABETES MEANS YOU'VE MESSED UP

Metformin tablets, prescribed to lower BG when a person has Type 2 diabetes, may only work in this capacity for a certain number of years before their effectiveness is reduced. When this happens, insulin is started to control BG levels instead. This is not a failure but the next necessary stage in the effective treatment of Type 2 diabetes.

Taking insulin does mean there is more likelihood of having a low BG and so more blood tests must be done each day – the up-side of this is that you will feel better as your BG control improves. Sometimes insulin is only needed temporarily because other illnesses stop BG-lowering tablets from working properly. It is also the case that with the availability of newer medications for Type 2 (these actually work better than insulin), people taking insulin can be switched to one of these (such as *rosiglitazone*) if Metformin stops working and insulin is started as an alternative.

Case Study

Kenny Walker found his Type 2 diabetes difficult to control. He weighed 14 stones, took 65 units of insulin daily and had an HbA1c level of 8% (65 mmol/L). His diabetes consultant decided to try rosagliazone to help Kenny's BG control by slowly introducing the medication while lowering his daily amount of insulin. Six months later Kenny was delighted to be told that he no longer needed to take insulin: he'd also lost nearly two stones in weight and his HbA1c level has come down to 6.5% (48 mmol/L).

Another point worth mentioning about Type 2 diabetes and insulin is that, for elderly people, the focus is NOT on the prevention of long-term complications such as eye and kidney disease which arise over a number of years due to continually high BG levels. This simplifies their diabetes management considerably as they do not have to worry about the potential consequences of poorer diabetes control.

PEOPLE WITH DIABETES CAN'T EXERCISE BECAUSE THEY'LL HAVE A HYPO

Any physical effort burns glucose in the muscles, so anything from ironing to hoovering or decorating will have an effect on your BG. The same goes for intense exercise – just ask former Olympic rower, Steve Redgrave, who has Type 1 diabetes. Intense activity can actually raise BG levels because the liver releases stored glucose to power the muscles. The key is anticipating glucose needs or potential BG increases and managing them so you don't get caught out.

Although it may seem like the most effort out of all the things people with diabetes are told they should be doing, moderate but regular exercise is a very good way to manage BG levels so they do not creep up. There are certain ways of exercising which are not advisable, like bouncing on a trampoline if you are susceptible to bleeds from the small blood vessels at the back of the eyes (*diabetic retinopathy*). It is also advisable that people with diabetic *neuropathy* (nerve damage) in their feet and those who are over 40 with diabetes seek medical advice before beginning an exercise programme. Your doctor will advise that you to start slowly and build up muscle strength, so don't go too mad too soon!

Case Study

Peter Dawson was 54 with Type 2 diabetes when he decided to buy a treadmill and get fit. He did not tell his diabetes consultant or his GP what he was planning, although both had advised him to take regular exercise to help manage his BG levels. After the machine was delivered to Peter's home he found the heavy exercise equipment strenuous to unpack, assemble, and drag into position where he wanted to use it. He then got onto the machine, set the pace button and began running without having exercised for many years. He had sudden pains in his chest and suffered a mild heart attack. His wife, Glynis called an ambulance and once Peter had undergone tests in hospital it was discovered that one of his coronary arteries was very narrow. He underwent treatment and now Peter still uses his treadmill, but on a much lower setting having been advised by the hospital physiotherapist about exercising safely following a heart attack. He is now doing well.

PEOPLE WITH DIABETES SHOULDN'T DRIVE

The key to driving safely is checking your BG levels before you set out. This is very important and I cannot stress enough that you must stop on long journeys to make sure your BG is not too low and not affecting your judgement (5.5 mmol/L and above suits me). The Driver and Vehicle Licensing Authority (DVLA) have to be informed if you develop Type 1 diabetes, or if you take insulin temporarily and have had a hypo. They must be told if there are any changes to your treatment or condition (such as numbness in the feet or sight complications). The DVLA will ask you to complete a questionnaire and have eye tests done to measure reaction times and peripheral vision every one, two or three years. There is one driving restriction – the DVLA does not allow people with Type 1 diabetes to drive a Large Goods Vehicle (LGV) or a Passenger Carrying Vehicle (PCV).

If you treat your diabetes with diet or diet and tablets you can hold a licence to drive a LGV or PCV. If you are not prescribed insulin you DO NOT have to inform the DVLA about your Type 2 diabetes, providing you have necessary eye checks and don't have hypos. They DO need to be told if you have had a hypo in the last 12 months and you needed the assistance of another person to treat it, or if you have reduced or absent hypo warning signs (*hypoglycaemia unawareness*) meaning you only know how low your glucose is by testing it rather than having any physical symptoms. In the United Stated driving laws for people with diabetes are different in every state and the American Diabetes Association provides details of these.

MUNG BEANS AND RED CABBAGE CAN CURE DIABETES
It is not surprising that people with diabetes want it to go away with as little effort as possible – I certainly do! There are any number of claims in the press and on the Internet about alternative therapies. Be warned of anything you read about diabetes on the Internet – unless it's on the Diabetes UK or American Diabetes Association website – suggesting that buying certain products will mean you can kiss goodbye to your unwanted condition.

I'm sure I don't need to say that you should be very cautious about following up on any of these claims that taking herbal concoctions makes diabetes go away – they're designed to gain the money of people with a serious health condition without any compassion or consideration for their health. Some of these pills are harmless, containing ingredients like powdered chalk, but others are made up of far more dangerous substances.

Basically I would advise that you only trust legitimate sources of information and tried and tested treatments provided by your diabetes health care team. There are medications such as aspirin that your GP may advise you take to thin your blood if you have diabetes, aiming to prevent blood clots forming in blood vessels. There is also a nutritional supplement called gingko biloba that can improve blood flow to the hands and feet but, alas, there is nothing you can take INSTEAD OF your insulin or BG-lowering medication.

A ROLLER COASTER OF EMOTINS

'I just felt like my body had let me down big-time…'

Everyone reacts differently to a diagnosis of diabetes – from total shock to feeling OK about the news because they know someone who has it, so they can see it is a manageable condition. Your own feelings about having diabetes will change over time as you begin to make sense of things, understand what having diabetes means and what you must do, and also when it all gets on top of you and you are just fed-up with it all. It's common to feel anger and stress when managing your diabetes, and at the beginning when you've just been told you have diabetes you may even try to ignore your diagnosis by being in denial.

Denial

Developing a serious health condition like diabetes can be like suffering a bereavement because it is the loss of your health, with similar feelings such as anger, denial, and depression before final acceptance of how your body, your health and your life has changed. This process can take a very long time to come to terms with, but diabetes doesn't give you that time.

As you may have already realised, being told you have diabetes is shocking and, whether you're ready to start dealing with it or not, suddenly there are all sorts of things you have to do and people you have to see.

Case Study

Chloe Parker was 20 when she was told she had Type 1 diabetes. She was also told that she would have diabetes for the rest of her life and that she would need to be careful of what she was eating and drinking, vigilantly counting carbohydrates and measuring insulin dosages; she was told to do regular BG tests – more if she took exercise, and to take more insulin when she was ill to prevent *hyperglycaemia* (high BG levels). She was sent on various carbohydrate-counting and diabetes self-management courses by her diabetes clinic. Four months after her diagnosis, Chloe had been admitted to hospital several times with dangerously high BG levels which led to *ketoacidosis* – a medical emergency. She was so overwhelmed by the massive change in her life she felt she couldn't cope. She just wanted it all to go away.

Case Study

Ravi Patel was told he had Type 2 diabetes when he was 44. He was in total shock and refused to believe the diagnosis because he hadn't actually been feeling ill, so it was a complete surprise. Before he'd even come to terms with the news, Ravi's GP had arranged for him to attend a diabetes education course (DESMOND – Diabetes Education and Self-Management for Ongoing and Newly Diagnosed) for people with Type 2 diabetes. Ravi went along to the course and, although there were other people like him also attending, he felt that he couldn't take all the information in. Ravi refused to accept that he would have to cut down on carbohydrate-rich foods so that his BG could be kept under control. Unfortunately, Ravi only went to part of the course. He had also not been taking the BG-lowering medication prescribed to him. He still has great trouble accepting the diagnosis.

This may sound familiar. Perhaps you find that even though you do all you can to manage your diabetes, BG levels are still not what both you and your health care team are aiming for so you just feel like giving up. This is because emotions play a huge role in BG fluctuations. Every person with diabetes experiences times when trying to manage this demanding condition day in, day out becomes all too much. This is NORMAL but obviously it's not a desirable or healthy situation to be in long-term, especially if not feeling able to manage diabetes becomes increasingly difficult due to other illnesses such as *depression*. I want to just say here that diabetes and depression often go hand in hand and it's common to feel depressed after diabetes is diagnosed.

FACT: Women with Type 2 diabetes are twice as likely than men with the condition to suffer from depression because of issues such as bodyweight and chronic complications.

You may feel that diabetes is a barrier to doing the things you want to do or being who you want to be, but this is absolutely not the case. Theresa May, Prime Minister of the United Kingdom, has Type 1 diabetes, as does the former Olympic rower Steve Redgrave, ex-professional footballer, Gary Mabbutt, and writer Anne Rice to name but a few. The list of famous people (past and present) with Type 2 diabetes is even longer and includes the likes of Elvis Presley, along with writers HG Wells and Ernest Hemmingway; the hugely successful film director, producer and screen writer, George Lucas; and the Oscar-winning actor, Tom Hanks. Actress, Halle Berry was initially diagnosed with Type 1 diabetes but it was then discovered that she actually has Type 2. The huge number of celebrities and famous people with diabetes goes to show that having the condition is certainly no barrier to achievement.

You may think that despite being given lots of information following your diagnosis, you don't know enough to be able to make alterations to your insulin regime for different life situations. This is only to be expected as you adjust to doing new things and coping with, for example, your first low BG level (*hypoglycaemia* or hypo for short). Fear of change and a sense of loss for the life you had before diabetes is also completely normal.

Blaming yourself for your diabetes

It is very common to feel that you have diabetes because of something you've done or not done, and this is especially the case if your child develops diabetes. There is absolutely nothing you could have done to prevent a diagnosis of Type 1 diabetes in either yourself or your child. When someone is diagnosed with Type 2 diabetes, blaming yourself is a very usual reaction, especially when you feel you haven't, perhaps, looked after yourself very well with the right foods or taking regular exercise.

It is true that being overweight, taking little or no exercise and smoking all contribute to poorer health, but big improvements in Type 2 diabetes and heart disease can be made by eating healthier foods, taking exercise several times a week and quitting smoking. Self-blame can lead to guilt and depression, so this is not a path to go down as it will prevent any focus on trying to improve health. Blame also stops you accepting that you have diabetes, although some people may find that blaming themselves helps motivate them to do some exercise or cut out junk food, helping them come to terms with their diagnosis.

FACT: Gaining an understanding of your diabetes and why it happened can actually give the condition meaning, helping you to cope and adapt to your diagnosis.

Case Study

Kunwarehanu Sandeep was diagnosed with Type 2 diabetes after having a routine blood test because his doctor thought he might be at risk. Kunwarehanu admits that he blames himself because he is several stones overweight, never does any exercise, eats junk food and smokes 30 cigarettes a day. Although his GP advised him to cut down on fatty foods and to try and walk to work three times a week instead of driving, Kunwarehanu has little enthusiasm for making improvements because he hasn't come to terms with his diabetes or how it may affect his life if he doesn't look after it. He has begun the process of change though by thinking about how he could alter his lifestyle in the future and do things differently.

Anxiety

After you are told you have diabetes it's common to feel anxious, and this can become debilitating if you feel like this for a long time. You may also have been feeling worried and anxious for quite a long time BEFORE your diabetes was diagnosed because you felt unwell for a while. You may have had concerns over certain symptoms, such as needing to visit the toilet more often and feeling thirsty, hoping they would go away. Anxiety may also have grown because you had to go to your doctor and you had to wait for your appointment, test results, and an answer to why you haven't felt right.

FACT: People with diabetes who are anxious tend to have higher BG results.

It's also natural to feel anxious because you expect to have to face lots of lifestyle changes once you know you have diabetes. This can be associated with the condition itself; your treatment and having to remember to take it on time; your BG results and whether they are too high or too low; needing to rely on health professionals to advise you; or when you don't get the information and support that you need from these people. These anxieties should become less as you learn to cope with your condition. Unfortunately, if your BG control is not good, you may become anxious about how diabetes will affect you over time, and about developing chronic complications of diabetes, especially if you have symptoms such as tingling in your feet, or blurred vision.

Case Study

Peter McKechnie developed Type 1 diabetes when he was 25. He felt this was incredibly inconvenient, disrupting his lifestyle and his plans. Peter resented his condition and begrudgingly did the absolute minimum to manage it by giving himself insulin twice a day and only testing his BG before bed. He was incredibly anxious about how having diabetes would affect his life: his future job prospects; travelling and going on holiday with his friends; whether he'd develop sight complications that would stop him driving; and needing to rely on other people if he had a serious hypo. Peter discussed these issues with a counsellor who was trained in dealing with people with chronic medical conditions and he eventually came to realise that the best thing he could do was take responsibility for his diabetes and to manage it as well as he could. This was because all the issues he was anxious about were more likely to happen if he had poor BG control, as this would increase his risk of complications and problems associated with his diabetes.

Anger

The majority of people with long-term (chronic) medical conditions feel angry, especially when it's a condition like diabetes that needs a great deal of self-care. Experts agree that anger comes from a build-up of physical energy (stress) that needs to be released from the body. Anger is triggered by frustration, tension, hostility, and irritation, and the way you cope with it is the key to stopping anger from damaging your health. Anger at a situation or another person creates negative thoughts because of YOUR PERCEPTION of that situation or that person's actions. As with all negative thoughts, it is a good idea to try and think through why they are in your mind and bothering you, and the same is true of angry emotions. You may not realise it, but there are three different kinds of anger:

- RAGE is explosive, violent, uncontrolled anger expressed as a destructive force.
- RESENTMENT is internal anger that boils away and is not unleashed on the person or object that's making you angry. It can bubble away for some time making you feel ill at ease and this is damaging both physically and psychologically.
- INDIGNATION is a more controlled form of anger, such as saying, 'How dare you!' to someone so they know they've overstepped the mark. It's far less destructive and perhaps the most positive form of anger.

Obviously when you're angry you don't stop and think about what form your anger should take as it's a defensive, reactionary emotion. Anger is therefore felt because someone or something has hurt you. Being diagnosed with diabetes can certainly cause anger for lots of reasons: your body has let you down; you now have a chronic medical condition; you have to look after diabetes as though it were a demanding child; you have to monitor what you eat and drink; you feel your diabetes stops you doing what you want to do; your family and friends don't understand diabetes or they make comments about you not looking after yourself properly; you can't manage your diabetes well, even though you try really hard; and so on and so on… What triggers your anger is a personal thing, but if you often feel angry, it's worth thinking about how to deal with it.

HOW DO I DEAL WITH ANGER?

It is best that you find a physical release for your anger, and by that I don't mean punching someone, however much satisfaction it might bring! It's important that you realise that you HAVE A CHOICE. You can throw a tantrum in the supermarket over the fact someone just ran over your foot with their trolley, or you can view the situation as an accident, be calm and accept that there's nothing you can do about it. Hopefully the person will apologise, but if they don't and burning resentment seethes through your whole body (it's happened to me more than once!), STAY IN CONTROL and tell yourself that the other person is rude and ill-mannered and then congratulate yourself for not losing your rag in public.

Physical exercise is a great way to reduce stress and anger – this can be by just by watching a boxing match on TV so that you don't have to get physically involved in the fight! If the situation that has made you angry has also made you very sad, a good cry can release the tension and the anger and you will feel so much better afterwards. Anger may also be controlled by labelling it as a person, so when you feel angry you say to yourself, 'Here's (insert a suitable name!) here to irritate and annoy me.' Other methods are counting out loud or shouting a word you have decided is your anger-word, such as, 'Oh, Rollocks' – (the things that hold the oars on a boat), or

'Pendulous Sedge!' (a plant found on river banks). People may stare, but it's better than shouting something far worse!

Guilt

Another strong emotion associated with the diagnosis of any health issue is that of guilt. This is especially related to thoughts of not having looked after yourself properly, or having done something wrong. Guilt also pops up every time you don't feel like exercising, if you eat something sweet, or if you realise you forgot to inject insulin or take glucose-reducing tablets at a certain time. Be assured – everyone with diabetes has done this at one time or another!

Feeling guilty is a negative emotion that can make diabetes self-management more difficult. Guilt is based on a feeling of unease due to bad behaviour – because you've done something wrong or you should have done something differently. It's also the feeling you get when you've been blaming yourself, for example, if you eat something 'naughty'. The guilt if you eat a cream cake is normal, but believing you are a bad person for doing so is negative and destructive.

When you have diabetes, guilt is an emotion you will often feel – from self-blame at developing the condition (and whether you could have prevented it in some way) to anger for having it, or developing complications because of it and feeling guilty that you could have done more to prevent them. Guilt also raises its head when you don't look after yourself as well as you know you should. It is completely NORMAL to feel guilty about aspects of diabetes and its care.

Case Study

Katriona Billings had great difficulty overcoming her sense of guilt when she developed Type 1 diabetes. She also had asthma and she'd read that the medication in her inhaler caused the pancreas to release insulin, so she felt she had, perhaps, taken too much of it, triggering her diabetes. The strong emotion of guilt exhausted her and made her lose her self-confidence. She also felt guilty for the worry and the burden she imagined she had put on her family and for resenting her happy, carefree friends who had no idea about diabetes or how it affected someone's life. When Katriona realised why she felt guilty she was able to challenge the emotion and reason with herself that it wasn't her fault – for developing Type 1 diabetes, or the fault of other people – the fact that they didn't have it and knew nothing about it. This helped Katriona to reduce her feelings of guilt and have more positive energy to spend on diabetes self-management activities.

HOW CAN I DEAL WITH MY FEELINGS OF GUILT?

- Focus on WHY you have feelings of guilt. Is it, for example, something you did or didn't do, or something someone else did that you know about and feel is wrong? Isolating the reason for guilt can make the situation feel less of a burden, or even make it go away completely.

- Share how you feel about your diabetes with others who are involved (if possible) and try to come up with a solution if there is anything that can be done. This might not be appropriate, but if you can begin to think in a more positive way it will reduce the guilty feelings.

- Don't cover up or try to ignore the guilt you feel you can't cope with as this will make it worse. It is also wise to avoid drinking and smoking more, or binge eating to try and take your mind off the guilt rather than facing it.

- Once you've identified the problem and a potential way of dealing with it (for example, that you often eat sweets because you need comfort but 'know you shouldn't'), contact a health professional who can offer you appropriate support and who you feel won't judge you. This might be your GP Practice Nurse, or Diabetes Nurse and this can help you devise ways of tackling the problem and the guilt you feel.

Stress

The word 'stress' can be used to mean anything from dealing with a difficult situation to the body's physical and mental reaction to everyday demands. We have to adapt ourselves to the situation we find ourselves in every day, whether that's a workman outside your house with a pneumatic drill, travelling on a very crowded train to work, a neighbour who just rubs us up the wrong way, or the stress involved in taking an exam. Whatever it is, it causes a *stress response* – something that makes our palms sweat, gives us heart palpitations, a headache, and or diahorrea, tightness in the throat, and makes us feel tense, agitated, nauseous, irritated, or short-tempered. Emotionally we are anxious, uneasy, worried, panic-stricken, angry, or frustrated.

HOW DOES STRESS AFFECT MY DIABETES?

When you are stressed and you have diabetes, the physical changes the body makes to deal with stress – releasing glucose to the muscles in the fight or flight response, and adrenaline to make sure we're alert – increases BG levels. This is harmful if you can't then burn this excess glucose off or reduce it with insulin. Other reactions to stress making your diabetes difficult to control are:

- An increase in blood flow to your muscles (taking glucose there to fuel them) which increases your blood pressure.
- Blood vessels are made smaller, increasing your heart rate, and breathing becomes rapid to supply more oxygen to all parts of the body.
- Digestion of food slows down as blood is taken away from this task and diverted to the muscles.
- You shake and sweat (like the symptoms of having a hypo). You may feel an adrenaline rush as it hurries through your system, and a headache may develop.
- Your mouth becomes dry and you feel sick.
- Muscles may become cramped and tight.

So, with all this going on, if you can't actually take your frustration out on the object causing you stress, or run away from something that is bothering you (like your boss), then the stress isn't released and it has no purpose in, or outlet from the body. This may cause even more stress and if it lasts over a period of time, this can severely affect the immune system so that serious illness occurs.

FACT: If the harmful imbalance in the body caused by stress continues over time this can lead to heart disease, hardening of the arteries, Type 2 diabetes, and certain types of cancer.

When stress affects us, the hormones that release stored glucose (*glycogen*) from the liver can't be used for energy when it enters the bloodstream without more insulin or BG-lowering medication. This increase in BG may also go undetected when you are stressed because you are preoccupied with the situation rather than regularly checking your BG levels. You also may not want to, or have time to eat or exercise, or you may choose to deal with the stress by drinking alcohol or smoking more than you usually do. You don't need me to tell you that these ways of 'coping' aren't particularly healthy ways of dealing with stress.

HOW CAN I DEAL WITH STRESS?

As you can see from the long list of ways stress affects the body, it is something that needs to be dealt with so that you are in control of your diabetes. There are several ways to help overcome the effects of stress on the body but you need to keep in mind:

FACT: Stress can be managed and controlled but it can't be totally removed.

- Use relaxation techniques such as deep breathing, meditation and hypnosis to reduce stress. This is effective because it allows your body to rest, especially if you haven't been sleeping well because of the situation that's causing your stress. It will also help you feel calmer and in control of the situation and of your diabetes, increasing your sense of wellbeing. You can also try (before you go to sleep) imagining that you are calm and stress-free, involving how each of your senses would react so, for example, you imagine that you are walking in a beautiful garden, planted with colourful and wonderfully-smelling flowers and you hear a waterfall nearby. This sort of imagery, if practised regularly, really can help reduce stress.

- Identify why you are feeling stressed. Knowing that the exact cause is (for example) trying to fit BG testing into a very busy lifestyle can help you to devise ways of dealing with it. Telling yourself you are just too busy to manage your diabetes during the day isn't specific enough – you need to know what the problem is to find a solution and reduce the stress.

- When you know what the problem is, the next thing to think about is how you react to that problem. I realised that I react before I've even fully assessed the situation and usually, things are not as bad as I've blown them up to be. Once I knew I was doing this, I was able to just take a breath when a stressful situation happens before flying off the handle.

  You can also deal with things that stress you by breaking them down into manageable parts so they don't seem such a big deal. You could also try identifying if you tend to react to stress physically (shouting and screaming) or emotionally (crying or worrying). When you know why and how you react, you can alter this response and, over time with repetition, your brain will automatically react in the way you want it to.

- Stay away from things that cause you stress as much as you possibly can. Obviously, if it's having diabetes itself that stresses you then you need to discuss better coping strategies with your diabetes team. If you can't avoid what stresses you, change the way you react by not responding negatively, i.e., saying or thinking, 'I knew this would happen to me, it always does,' or, 'I bet no one else has these problems – I'm such a loser.'

- Exercise, as I've previously mentioned, is not only a good way of reducing your BG levels, it also helps to relieve stress. The best exercise is ENJOYABLE EXERCISE, like swimming, dancing, or brisk walking, for example, to help release tension.

- Take up a hobby or leisure activity you enjoy to help relieve your stress. It's a diversion and stops you thinking about the situation. If it's a productive hobby, like writing, the creation of something new can be motivating and is also very therapeutic if you can get your emotions and feeling down on paper (or a computer screen).

- Try to get as much sleep as you can if stress has been preventing you from getting a good night's rest. Even if you end up having a sleep because you're tired and it's not bed-time, this is because your body needs it to relax and repair itself.

Fear

It is completely natural to be fearful when you are told you have diabetes, and for what lies ahead when you've had it for some time. You may not think of questions to ask about diabetes until after the news has sunk in, or feel you can't ask something because it seems like a silly question. All the issues surrounding diabetes as a chronic condition can lead to fear of the unknown.

FACT: Fear of needles is very common for people with and without diabetes.

Obviously, if you have to take insulin to treat your diabetes, having a fear of needles can make this difficult. There are options available if this applies to you so you can inject without seeing the needle. Many people say that it's a fear of what's going to happen rather than the actual process or any pain that might happen at the time. Insulin pump therapy (where a small plastic tube, or *cannula*, is placed under the skin so insulin can be delivered as required) is also an option for people with needle phobia. This is especially helpful if you currently have to take multiple daily injections (MDI) of insulin. Your diabetes team will be able to arrange this if appropriate, or show you how to inject insulin as quickly and painlessly as possible.

When you have had diabetes for a little while the questions you have may be answered in the course of time, but this doesn't mean that the fear goes away, for example, 'Will I develop complications?' You may worry about this for many years and, if they do develop, fear of how they will progress may be what worries you. Because it's drummed into us from diagnosis, a fear of developing chronic diabetic complications like eye and kidney disease is very common. This type of fear is to be expected, but living in a permanent state of fearfulness is not healthy for you or your diabetes.

Obviously the best way to overcome a fear of complications is to control your diabetes as well as you possibly can and keep BG levels within normal limits. The way to deal with diabetes-related fear is to plan for situations BEFORE they happen. Below are some ways to overcome general fears associated with your diabetes:

- You may fear that you won't be able to cope with having diabetes because it's too difficult and that potential problems will be impossible to overcome. The best way to deal with this is to write down the things that you fear about diabetes self-management and then find solutions such as speaking to your diabetes nurse. If you fear night-time hypoglycaemia and you live alone, for example, this can be helped with a continuous glucose sensor that alerts you with an alarm to wake you when your BG falls below a certain safe limit, such as 4 mmol/L.

- Remind yourself that chronic complications do not inevitably happen when you have diabetes. If you do develop MILD neuropathy (nerve damage) in your feet, mild nephropathy in your kidneys, or mild retinopathy in your eyes, the effects are not severe and you can still live your life the way you want to.

- Use the fear of complications to motivate you to manage your diabetes in the best way you can to keep your HbA1c levels (the glucose sticking to the red blood cells) low.

- If you have had diabetes for a number of years and you have complications that now limit you, concentrate on the things you can still do. You may not (for example) be able to drive anymore because of sight problems but you may (for example) be able to draw or paint.

- Don't dwell on feeling like you're a burden on your family and friends when you need some help with daily tasks because of long-term complications. The people closest to you like to be involved in helping you with your diabetes as it makes them feel needed and useful!

- You may fear pain in relation to complications. Peripheral neuropathy (burning and needle-like pains in the feet or hands) can be painful, but there are medications that can treat this (*Gabapentin* and *Memantine*). Other complications, such as *autonomic neuropathy* (damage to the nerves controlling functions like digestion and heartbeat), nephropathy (kidney disease), and retinopathy (eye disease) ARE NOT painful conditions. Everyone with diabetes, as with the non-diabetic population, gets a twinge of pain now and then so try not to fear that something serious is going on with your diabetes.

- Some people fear how other people will react – are you worried about telling people you have diabetes? So many people have the condition now (one in four) that it's not something to worry about. Diabetes ISN'T CATCHING, so people won't avoid you if you tell them. The response I usually get is, 'Oh, my mother or father or sister or brother or son or daughter or aunty or uncle has that!', or EVEN, 'So do I!'

- If you feel that you have to tell someone important about your diabetes, such as your boss, and you fear how he/she will react, then you must find the easiest way of doing this. YOU DON'T HAVE to tell an employer that you have diabetes unless they ask any medical questions, but you may want to tell them anyway so they know what to do if you have a hypo at work.

- Don't fear travelling to other countries if you have diabetes. It's such a widespread condition globally now that hospitals, clinics and pharmacies will be aware of what you need if you become ill, or run out of your medication. If you fear that you don't speak the language of the country you're visiting, invest in a phrase book so you can make yourself understood and familiarise yourself with key words before you go.

Plan your trip carefully and make sure you take extra medication and supplies with you. If it's a hot country you are visiting, you can buy a cooler bag to put your insulin in as HEAT DEGRADES INSULIN as it's a protein (think of how cheese changes when you grill it). Check on the Internet or with your travel agent before you leave to find out where the nearest medical facilities are to where you'll be staying to give you some peace of mind.

FACT: By facing the things about diabetes that you're afraid of, whether physically doing them or mentally identifying them, you can reduce and even get rid of the fear.

Case Study

Mauro Pelargrino was told he had Type 2 diabetes after having a routine blood test at his GP surgery. He felt alone and isolated, but most of all, he felt fear. His GP suggested he go along to a local diabetes support group where he could meet and speak to other people with the condition and discus how he felt. Mauro didn't really want to go along and sit in a roomful of people with diabetes because he felt they wouldn't understand his fear, and that they would all be old hands at managing the condition. After Mauro had been to a few meetings he realised that everyone else was struggling with the same issues as he was, and he admits he learned lots of ways to help himself to manage his diabetes.

Coping Strategies

Coping with the diagnosis of any chronic condition is similar to coping with a very stressful event because we must adapt and cope with a long-term negative change in lifestyle that wasn't expected, wanted or planned for. If the way you usually cope with stressful events is to try and ignore them, this won't work with diabetes as it will cause you more problems in the long run.

Other reactions that some people have are blaming someone else for their diabetes, treating it as thoug it's not a big deal, and letting the diagnosis wash over them without responding to what they're told. These forms of 'coping' result in poor BG control. Those people who take the news seriously but don't react with distress tend to deal with the management of their diabetes very well.

Case Study

Ana Blake was shocked when she was first told that she had Type 2 diabetes but she quickly realised that this was something she needed to get on top of. She read as much as she could about how to manage the condition because she was curious, and found that this actually helped her to accept her diagnosis and begin to manage it properly. Diabetes wasn't something that she wanted in her life, but Ana realised that the news had to be faced up to or else the situation would become worse.

Relief

It may sound strange, but many people are actually relieved when they finally get a diagnosis and an explanation of their symptoms, especially if they knew something was wrong. As we've already seen, the symptoms of diabetes can be very different from person to person. For this reason, knowing that diabetes is the reason for certain symptoms helps provide hope that insulin or BG-reducing medication will control these symptoms and improve wellbeing for the better.

There are people who try to put on a brave face or make excuses for the symptoms of diabetes, such as that they're due to the pressures of work, getting older, or even that they're just imagining having to go to the toilet more often because they're drinking more cups of tea every day. This is a form of denial and it acts as a protection measure rather than admitting that there is something wrong. Finding out that there is a genuine physical reason for the symptoms helps the individual realise it wasn't 'all in their head'.

Case Study

Andy Cowling was 60 and had been feeling tired for a long time. He put it down to getting older and, perhaps, not getting enough iron in his diet, imagining that he might be anaemic. Andy bought himself some iron supplements from the chemist, but after three months, there was no improvement and he still felt tired. Andy then thought he must be imagining feeling tired because it was to be expected in a man of his age – needing a nap mid-afternoon and a second cup of tea after each meal as his mouth was dry. This went on for a year and a half until finally, Andy had to go to the dentist and she told him that he should visit his GP for a BG test. Andy followed his dentist's advice and discovered that he had Type 2 diabetes a week layer. He felt a huge sense of relief when he received the diagnosis, realising that he had a reason for his tiredness and thirst. He also felt daft that he hadn't wanted to make a fuss!

Changing moods and emotions

How you feel can be down to your BG being too low or too high: mood swings are also very normal in people with diabetes because of this. Your brain needs a constant supply of glucose to function properly, so if your BG is low you become irritable, depressed, tired, short-tempered and upset. The effects of high and low BG on the brain appear as very similar symptoms and sometimes it's difficult to know if you're high or low without testing your BG to find out. You may not even connect being angry or irritated with your BG – it took me some years to recognise this as I just thought I had a short fuse and little patience! Having a high level of available glucose does not, as you would expect, make your brain work better. It actually irritates it because too much glucose is a toxin.

High BG levels make you feel irritated, on edge, frustrated, annoyed, and even vicious. I have been known to say horrible things to loved ones when I'm too high (or low) and, not withstanding how they have to develop a thick skin and understand that you don't mean it, you are left with feelings of guilt afterwards for 'being moody'. It's a difficult one because at some stage your personality will be temporarily altered by your BG and explaining this to those around you can be hard.

Case Study

Sally Morris had very difficult to control Type 1 diabetes meaning that her BG levels would swing from high to low without warning – something she found hard to cope with. Her husband Gary was used to the situation and didn't take the things Sally said to heart, such as her shouting that he should leave her alone when he was trying to help reverse her hypoglycaemia with sweet tea. Gary would assure Sally that her moods were not her fault. One day Gary's parents came to stay and Sally had a bad hypo followed by hyperglycaemia because her liver had released stored glucose – Sally was battling to bring it down again. Gary's parents didn't understand the situation and had never seen Sally act in this snappy and sarcastic way before. Sally later overheard her mother-in-law describing her as hostile. This upset Sally greatly and she was overwhelmed with a sense that people just didn't understand. She decided to apologise, although she strongly felt she shouldn't have to. When she said sorry she expected her parents-in-law to understand that it was her BG levels but instead they said, 'We don't know why you had to act like that.' Sally was angry at the injustice for a long time afterwards and felt isolated by the experience.

I will repeat that it is perfectly normal to feel overwhelmed by a diagnosis of diabetes and trying to meet the daily demands necessary to manage the condition well. Many people find they have difficulties with adopting lots of new behaviours in their life – taking insulin or medication in the right dose at the right time, doing regular blood tests throughout the day, weighing or carbohydrate-counting foods, keeping active, attending various hospital clinics and GP checks, and so on. Self-care habits such as these take months, if not longer to become the sorts of things you do without thinking each day. Think how often you had to be reminded to clean your teeth as a child before you did it automatically!

A much easier way around having to do new self-care tasks is to take one thing at a time. Obviously some things take priority, such the need for daily insulin or BG-lowering medication and blood tests, but if you set your own priorities to get to grips with something new that you feel is a realistic goal, it is an achievement when you master it. This also means you are less likely to go back to your old ways. I have though, known people who say that they sometimes forget to do their insulin injections after 20 years of having Type 1 diabetes. They only realise when they eat and feel very sick about an hour afterwards because their BG is sky high. This goes to show that even the most experienced person with diabetes can still slip up sometimes – me included, and on more than one occasion. BUT not to do the same thing again.

FACT: The way you feel – mental health – is just as important as physical health.

Understanding how your emotions affect your diabetes is the key to coming to terms with the condition and being able to manage these ups and downs so that you are in control of your diabetes rather than it being in control of you. One key way of being in control is having what is called *self-efficacy* – the self-confidence to do things, like using a BG testing machine, or drawing up and injecting insulin, and building on that to know you can tackle similar challenges. I recently had to start using a new *insulin pump* (a piece of technology that delivers insulin continuously under the skin). I will be completely honest – I had to force myself to get acquainted with it because it was different to what I'm used to. It was the same principle as the pumps I'd used for the past 16 years, but it reminded me that with diabetes, you never stop learning.

Other people can also be very good at making you feel bad unintentionally because they want the best for you. Because diabetes is the only chronic condition where the person who has it provides 95% of their own care (as opposed to nurses or doctors) other people's comments are an area that often requires a thick skin. Most people are only being kind, but strangers can sometimes come out with something thoughtless.

I was once at the Science Museum in London and visited the facilities to test my BG and inject some insulin (before I used an insulin pump). The bathroom was empty so I washed my hands and got on with it. I could have gone into a cubicle, but I always question the hygiene aspect of doing this. A woman then burst in, stared open-mouthed in disbelief as I injected my upper arm flesh, and she retreated back into the museum shouting, 'There's a druggie in the toilets!' How embarrassing (cringe!)

Case Study

Colin Stoddard was diagnosed with Type 2 diabetes over ten years ago but felt that other people were the biggest problem for him. It seemed that wherever he went people assumed they knew more about his condition than he did, or that they were interfering in his life. At work colleagues would say things like, 'Should you be eating that?' when Colin's BG was low and he was eating a biscuit with his morning coffee. At home his wife would often suggest that he should be walking the dog or gardening to get some exercise, and if he went to his daughter's house for Sunday lunch, she would control Colin's food portions rather than letting his chose for himself. Over the years these small annoyances built up into major irritations and in the end, Colin told people that he would make his own decisions, thank you very much. He then felt guilty because he knew everyone was just looking out for him. He just couldn't win!

Hopefully you won't experience too many thoughtless comments from strangers, but 'advice' from friends, family and work mates is very common. The more you actively learn about your diabetes the better. TAKE YOUR TIME AND GO AT YOUR OWN PACE. I won't lie, IT IS a steep learning curve, but the more you find out about up-to-date and reliable diabetes information, education and support, the less likely you are to worry: a better understanding means you can manage the condition effectively.

FACT: Feeling diabetes-related guilt is like taking your diabetes medication – it's an integral part of the condition.

Depression

Although they are two separate conditions, depression does develop more often in people with diabetes, and Type 2 diabetes can develop following a period of depression. Both depression and diabetes can be isolating and cause you to think that no one understands or that you just want to give up. This can be the case if you're trying hard to do your best but your BG levels don't show that. As we've already seen, many things affect your diabetes control, such as stress which can increase BG due to hormonal variations that make the liver release stored glucose. Stress may occur as a result of feeling in denial about your diagnosis and in association with feelings of anger, but it's important not to let this manifest as ignoring the need for insulin or tablets.

FACT: Depression affects at least 15% of people with diabetes and can have an adverse effect on BG control, diabetes self-management and chronic complications in both adults and children.

Case Study

Sylvia Walker felt her life was over when she was diagnosed with diabetes. She felt she was no use to anyone and that her efforts to control her Type 2 diabetes were useless. Sylvia felt so low she wondered why she was even bothering at all as it was 'only Type 2' and, in her eyes, not as serious as the Type 1 diabetes affecting one of her relatives. She reasoned that as her diabetes was causing her to feel so bad psychologically, if she just didn't think about it then maybe her life could go back to the way it was? Sylvia's GP prescribed anti-depressants to try and lift her mood and she is currently waiting to see a counsellor who specialises in depression and health issues.

Depression is three times more likely to occur in people with diabetes and this is a problem because it not only impacts on mental health but in terms of diabetes, it also affects a person's ability to self-manage their condition. This, in turn, leads to poor BG control which can trigger chronic complications over time.

FACT: Although depression is a major issue for people with diabetes it is often not diagnosed, especially if the person doesn't tell their GP, Practice Nurse or diabetes team how they feel.

WHAT ARE THE SYMPTOMS OF DEPRESSION?
There are many symptoms of depression, such as:
- Feeling very sad, unmotivated or dejected.
- Loss of appetite that is not because of high BG levels or your diabetes medication.
- Being unable to sleep because sad thoughts keep running through your mind.
- Sleeping too much because that way, you can switch your mind off.
- Withdrawing from the social events you enjoy.
- Crying for no particular reason, especially if this is unlike you.
- Focusing on things that happened in the past that you can do nothing about.
- Feeling hopeless, inadequate or worthless.
- Often feeling angry and very irritable when it's not because of your BG levels.

- Feeling more fearful of situations.
- Having little interest in work, family, or other interests or lacking concentration.
- Having little energy, but not if this is due to your BG or other health issues.
- Thinking, speaking or acting in a more reserved way than normal.

The more of these symptoms that you recognise in you or another person with diabetes, the more likely you/they are to have depression.

HOW CAN I HELP MYSELF?

The best thing you can do to keep depression at bay or under control if you already have it is to make sure your BG levels are within normal limits of 5–7 mmol/L. This is because hormonal and chemical changes that occur in the body with depression act to increase BG levels and so, even if you don't feel like eating (or haven't eaten) anything, your BG may still be very high.

FACT: Depression interacts negatively with diabetes, leading to unpredictable diabetes control and a 1.8% increase in HbA1c.

There are other things you can do as well as keeping tight control of your BG to help fight depression. Focusing on accomplishing a long-term goal that you have can really help to reduce depressive symptoms as it takes a lot of energy to be depressed – by diverting your attention, your brain is dealing with reaching your goal and not generating depressed feelings. Similarly, keeping yourself physically active not only helps to reduce your BG, it also helps release anger, irritations and frustrations if you chose an activity that makes you feel positive by releasing 'feel-good' hormones (*endorphins*). Don't forget to speak to your GP or diabetes care team about the RIGHT SORT of exercise for you before you go off and start pounding a punch bag at the gym!

It is also important to realise the times when you are thinking in a negative way. Ask yourself, what set it off? What were you thinking about before you began to feel miserable? It's obviously not good to be thinking negative thoughts, so can you actually divide the problem into things you can do something about, like being overweight and being able to change this situation, or are they things you have no control over?

If this is the case then realising you can do nothing, (for example, the death of a loved one), and that you can't turn back the clock can be a revelation. If the situation(s) that are making you depressed are ones you can't do anything about, then you have to let it go. It's the THOUGHT of these things that has triggered your negative emotions so try to catch yourself going down this path and change your thought patterns – think of an occasion when you were really happy and remember how you felt.

Emotions are constantly changing so what you feel and think isn't lasting. I've noticed that I can be incredibly down one day and positive and joking the next. The key is NOTICING your mood so you can know why you're thinking a certain way. It really does help to deal with depression over time.

Another thing I've realised more and more lately is that everyone has something to worry about in their life, so trying to see things from another person's perspective can help you see why they react in a certain way. Often we don't know what others have to cope with. As with the example of the friend with the unwell child, negative thoughts can lead to negative actions. I have actually imagined that someone has slighted me when I'm depressed and told myself I wouldn't bother with them again, only to find later that I'd got it completely wrong. Beware of acting rashly when you are depressed because you may have misread the situation. Negative thoughts and actions can also lead to deeper depression, so trying to recognise and break this cycle is important. NEGATIVE THOUGHTS ARE NOT GOOD FOR YOUR DIABETES CONTROL!

Share your feelings, thoughts and worries with other people who will listen and care (i.e., not a random stranger on the bus or in the doctor's surgery who will shrug their shoulders and make you feel worse). Make sure you tell your diabetes team how you feel as they may be able to refer you to a specialist psychologist or counsellor who can help resolve the issues causing your depression. It may also be the case that your depression is caused by a chemical imbalance or deficiency, so if it lasts for a long time, even after treatment with anti-depressant medication or therapy, this may be the reason and it can be treated.

FACT: If someone doesn't like the fact you have diabetes then you don't need them in your life!

Relationships

PARTNERS AND GOOD FRIENDS

When you have diabetes it can be difficult to know when to introduce this into a conversation with a new partner (or friend). You may imagine that your new soul mate will go running for the hills if you introduce diabetes into the conversation, and this can make you nervous about telling them and especially how to explain it.

Most people have heard of diabetes before, but as my husband told me when I first brought the subject up, he didn't really know much about it – other than that it was something to do with sugar. Don't expect people to automatically understand what you're telling them about your diabetes. BUT If someone is truly interested in you as a person, the fact you have diabetes won't put them off!

> Case Study
>
> Lee Brown was 19 when he met his girlfriend, Annie. After a few dates he became more and more worried that telling her he had diabetes would put her off. Lee's mum, Linda, told him he should just explain the facts simply, making sure he mentioned how low BG levels could affect him and how Annie could help. When Lee plucked up the courage to let Annie know he explained the basics of the condition, hypo warning signs and how to treat it quickly. She listened carefully and then asked sensible questions. This made Lee realise that Annie was actually interested in his diabetes – she wanted to know as much as possible. Two years on they are now engaged, have bought a house together and hope to marry later this year.

As you've already seen, emotions and diabetes go hand in hand and the people closest to you need to be told (although they probably have already noticed!) how you act when you are feeling horrible because your BG is too low or too high. They will also soon realise if they know you fairly well (although it doesn't hurt to mention it to people you care about) that you will be your usual self again once your BG is back within normal range.

Don't ever feel that you have to cover your diabetes up: everyone you meet has usually had some kind of medical history – from an ingrown toenail to arthritis. In the case of diabetes, it's telling people if you need to eat, do an injection, do a blood test, feel low – whatever. People DO generally understand (with the exception of that woman in the Science Museum toilets) and they are usually interested in finding out more. This might annoy the heck out of you, but see it as an opportunity to educate others about what you have to do every day to keep well.

I will hold up my hands and say I was guilty of trying to IGNORE MY DIABETES when I was in my teens. I never did a blood test and I didn't pay particular attention to eating properly or regularly and this went on until I was in my twenties and met my husband. This behaviour has severely bitten me on the bottom in later years. I have spoken to many people who feel the same about their diabetes – if only they could turn back the clock with their current knowledge and do things differently. I will talk about how you can avoid developing the chronic complications of diabetes in the next chapter.

HOW WILL DIABETES AFFECT ME?

'I know that managing diabetes is a head to toe problem'

Blood glucose levels are continually fluctuating up and down, especially when you eat. This is why you will be told to measure your BG levels often throughout the day and sometimes during the night, and even more often if you develop an infection (like a cold or flu) or when you exercise. How often you should test your BG is determined by the kind of diabetes you have, the treatment you take for it, and how well that treatment manages your condition to keep it stable. Variations in BG, as we've just seen, can have an enormous effect on personality and mood. This is not our fault or something we can control (we are not consciously being bad-tempered and irritable) but trying to keep BG within normal limits allows the brain to function correctly without irritation from very high glucose levels, or to go into panic and shock from very low levels.

Hospital blood tests

The blood tests you do yourself at home are the best way of showing you what your BG is at that moment in time and what you need to do next, but they don't tell you how good your overall diabetes self-management is over, say, several months. When you have an HbA1c test done at the hospital or a blood testing clinic a sample of blood is taken from a vein to see how much glucose has stuck to the red blood cells over a three-month period. This is because red blood cells are renewed every three months, so you won't be asked to have this test done any more frequently than this while your diabetes is being stabilised and your consultant reviews how well your treatment is working. Once your diabetes is under control you will have an HbA1c blood test usually once every six-months to a year for your annual diabetes review.

The Powers That Be decided a few years ago to stop measuring HbA1c as a percentage concentration of glucose in the blood over time and began measuring it in millimoles per litre (mmol/L) in the same was as home blood testing machines do. I personally prefer the old-fashioned percentage measurement of HbA1c as an indicator of how good my BG control has been, as do many diabetes specialists, but the modern way doesn't agree with me. I've provided a table below to show how HbA1c percentage converts to mmol/L and vice versa so you can judge how good your glucose control has been. You may also find this table useful if you read books and articles about diabetes published a few years ago that have used percentage HbA1c values.

Case Study

Angela White was planning to become pregnant and was advised by her GP to tighten her BG control as much as she could manage to make sure she was as healthy as possible before conception. Her HbA1c had been 7.2% (55 mmol/L) but her GP suggested she aim for 6–6.5% (42–48 mmol/L). Angela was motivated to test her BG more frequently and to exercise after meals to stop any sharp increases in BG. When she had her next HbA1c test three months later she had achieved her goal and, by keeping a close eye on her BG levels, she went on to have a healthy pregnancy and a normal weight healthy baby girl. Because Angela had made the lifestyle changes of exercising after meals and checking her BG often for the sake of her baby and had done this for a year, she continues to do this as she had more energy.

HbA1c %	mmol/L	HbA1c %	mmol/L	HbA1c %	mmol/L	HbA1c %	mmol/L
4.0	20	6.0	42	8.0	64	10.0	86
4.1	21	6.1	43	8.1	65	10.1	87
4.2	22	6.2	44	8.2	66	10.2	88
4.3	23	6.3	45	8.3	67	10.3	89
4.4	25	6.4	46	8.4	68	10.4	90
4.5	26	6.5	48	8.5	69	10.5	91
4.6	27	6.6	49	8.6	70	10.6	92
4.7	28	6.7	50	8.7	72	10.7	93
4.8	29	6.8	51	8.8	73	10.8	95
4.9	30	6.9	52	8.9	74	10.9	96
5.0	31	7.0	53	9.0	75	11.0	97
5.1	32	7.1	54	9.1	76	11.1	98
5.2	33	7.2	55	9.2	77	11.2	99
5.3	34	7.3	56	9.3	78	11.3	100
5.4	36	7.4	57	9.4	79	11.4	101
5.5	37	7.5	58	9.5	80	11.5	102
5.6	38	7.6	60	9.6	81	11.6	103
5.7	39	7.7	61	9.7	83	11.7	104
5.8	40	7.8	62	9.8	84	11.8	105
5.9	41	7.9	63	9.9	85	11.9	107

Knowing your HbA1c can help you to plan and achieve a healthy pregnancy, and to give you more energy because your body is not having to cope with high glucose levels that make you feel sluggish. By maintaining normal BG levels throughout pregnancy, this allows the baby's nervous system and organs to develop correctly and for the baby to be a healthy weight when it's born.

Your own BG monitoring tests

Forgive me for stating the obvious, but the reason you need to check your BG levels regularly is to find out if you have too much or too little insulin or glucose-lowering medication working at certain times of the day and night. If there is too little insulin, your BG levels will be high; too much insulin and your BG will be low.

HIGH BLOOD GLUCOSE (HYPERGLYCAEMIA)

HYPERGLYCAEMIA is the medical term for high blood glucose levels. As you know, when there is a lack of insulin, or it can't be used properly by the body, high BG levels are the result (as a basic rule this means glucose meter readings in double figures). If this situation lasts over a period of time, like when you have a bad cold, the excess glucose causes the blood to become acidic and if too little insulin is available, this becomes a medical emergency known as *diabetic ketoacidosis* (DKA) needing hospital attention. When ketoacidosis happens your body doesn't have enough insulin (or BG-lowering medication) to work properly. Instead of being able to use glucose for fuel, when there is not enough insulin your body has to switch to using fat and protein for energy meaning it can even break down muscle instead. The acid by-products of this break down are called *ketones* – hence diabetic ketoacidosis.

FACT: Making sure you do more BG tests when you are ill – increasing insulin dosages to avoid hyperglycaemia can keep you out of hospital as you will be reducing your risk of diabetic ketoacidosis.

CAUSES OF DIABETIC KETOACIDOSIS

- Under-dosing or deliberate repeated omission of insulin – your body can't go without insulin for long as it is needed to convert starch and glucose into energy.
- Any kind of infection that increases BG levels so that you need more insulin.
- Physical or emotional trauma.

- Heart attack.

- Alcohol and/or drug abuse, particularly cocaine.

- Medications such as corticosteroids (these come as tablets/inhalers/injections and creams used to treat inflammation), and diuretics (water tablets).

SYMPTOMS OF DKA

- Sickness and vomiting – this happens because of the build-up of acids from the breakdown of fat and protein used for fuel and because your body is lacking certain chemicals.

- Rapid breathing (known *as Kussmaul breathing*) – this happens when your blood is very acidic and your body tries to pant some of this acid out. The breath of a person with DKA often smells like acetone (nail polish remover) or pear drops.

- Tiredness and lethargy – this happens because your body can't use glucose for fuel when your BG is very high. Your brain is trying to work as normal with thick, syrupy blood lacking in essential nutrients when you have ketoacidosis.

- Weakness in the muscles – again, this happens because your body can't use glucose as fuel for muscle function and it begins to break down fat and then protein in the muscles instead.

Case Study

Michael Barlow was 18, had Type 1 diabetes and was always getting colds and sore throats because of his weakened immune system. His diabetes consultant and GP told him to look after himself properly when he was ill, but he didn't know what that meant, other than that he should rest. When Michael felt another cold coming on he bought a carton of orange juice and drank it in the belief he was doing himself good. Two days later he was admitted to hospital with a BG level of 25.2 mmol/L and a high level of ketones in his urine. Michael was put on an insulin drip and was told that he should have monitored his BG levels every two or three hours, increased his insulin by one-third to cover the extra glucose produced during an infection, and that the high amount of fruit sugar in the orange juice he was drinking had caused his ketoacidosis to be more serious by increasing his BG.

FACT: Diabulimia – deliberately under-dosing on insulin to lose weight – occurs in 1 in every 400 males and 1 in every 50 females; this is one-third of all adults taking insulin. This means additional admissions to hospital with DKA for these people as they are not taking enough insulin.

TREATMENT OF DKA

Diabetic ketoacidosis is classed as a medical emergency. If you have to be admitted to hospital with DKA you should understand the treatment you will receive so you know what to expect. Because there is a chemical imbalance in your body, your system will be acidic and lacking water as high BG levels cause excretion of more urine to flush out glucose and ketone by-products from the break-down of fat and protein. Health professionals aim to provide treatment to reduce the acidity level of your blood, replace the level of *potassium* that is lost, and to stabilise BG back down to normal levels.

Each of these levels will be regularly measured by hospital staff and charted so a record can be kept of improvements. You will be put onto an intravenous drip to give a large quantity of vital fluids:

potassium, insulin and other necessary medications. Because the body responds very well to the insulin that it needs so badly, BG levels stabilise quickly and may even reach hypo levels. This will be detected quickly by regular BG tests and the insulin in the drip may be replaced by a glucose/insulin solution. Once BG goes back down to stable levels, your body will begin to work normally again, stopping the breakdown of fat and protein for fuel. Ketones in the blood from the breakdown of fat and protein will be excreted from the body.

As your body recovers and chemical balance is restored you will stop feeling and being sick and your brain will be able to function properly so mental functioning will return to normal. Nursing staff will encourage you to take sips of water to make sure the stomach can tolerate it and, as long as you are not sick, you will be allowed to drink water and eat solid food. When the doctor caring for you feels you have recovered your intravenous drip will be removed and you'll be able to start injecting insulin again.

LOW BLOOD GLUCOSE (HYPOGLYCAEMIA)
If you have diabetes, having a hypo (low BG) is something you will experience from time to time. HYPOGLYCAEMIA is the medical term for low blood glucose. Low BG levels of 4 mmol/L or less in people with diabetes can be due to an excess of insulin or BG-lowering medication and not enough available glucose. Hypoglycaemia can happen because of the timing of your insulin injections or medication – the food you eat may not be digested at the same time as the insulin or medication is working. You may then have a high BG later on because the food is now digested but there

is not enough insulin available as it's already stopped working. If you are having hypos before meals and high BG readings later on this is probably what's happening.

FACT: Always treat hypoglycaemia as soon as possible with glucose tablets so that this can be quickly absorbed into your bloodstream to increase low glucose levels. Eating something sweet if you don't have glucose tablets may take longer to work as your body has to break down the food to be able to use the glucose.

FACT: If you tend to have severe hypos where your BG drops very low (and you pass out) you need to have a Glucagen injection kit in the house and for another person to know where it is and how to use it. If you don't recover, or have a second hypo after Glucagen is given, an ambulance is needed so they can give you intravenous glucose.

Although you can't always stop a hypo from happening, you can control it by taking action quickly. You should speak to your diabetes nurse or consultant so they can advise you about how to make the correct adjustments in the timing of your medication dosages. Here's a few other reasons why your BG might drop:

MEDICATION

If you have changed the dose of insulin or BG-lowering medication (for example, if your diabetes consultant has advised that you to increase it, or you've found you need more insulin at certain times of the day) you may have more hypos. The timing of your injections or tablets may also be the reason, as it's doing its job to lower BG when there's no food for it to work on. Remember that different types of insulin work at different times, so make sure you know when yours has its peak working time – the time you are most likely to have a hypo if there's not enough food available. If you miss a meal or take your insulin too early, your BG level will become low. If you take sulphonylurea medication for Type 2 diabetes and you are eating less, your medication will need to be reduced. If you take sulphonylureas or a combination of diabetes medication that includes sulphonylureas, these can cause hypoglycaemia. Eat a snack mid-morning and mid-afternoon to avoid low BG at these times and tell your diabetes nurse or Practice nurse about this.

EXERCISE

If you take moderate exercise for 20–45 minutes three times a week that DOESN'T get you out of breath this is not only good for your heart; doing this for 20–30 minutes a day can also help you to control your BG levels after meals. When you exercise in a moderate, paced way it generally burns BG and this means you may become hypo. If you plan to take _moderate_ exercise you should lower your insulin or increase your carbohydrate intake so that you don't become low during or afterwards. It is also possible to use exercise to manage your BG levels and avoid taking extra insulin if, for example, your BG is slightly raised to 10 mmol/L when you want to be 6 mmol/L.

FACT: MODERATE EXERCISE means different things to different people. If you haven't exercised regularly, cycling very slowly on an exercise bike is moderate while for others, it might be jogging. **REMEMBER** – it's moderate if it <u>doesn't</u> get you out of breath.

- Build up your exercise endurance to steadily improve your cardiovascular health.
- Do exercises regularly that strengthen your muscles and build up muscular endurance so that your body benefits from the effort and you feel fitter and healthier. (Muscles, ligaments and tendons become shorter over time with diabetes).
- Aim to increase how flexible you are by setting goals – if you want to be able to touch your toes, for example.
- If you are overweight, chose exercises that burn body fat such as swimming, cycling or using a treadmill.

The good news is, the more you weigh, the more calories you burn off just for your body to function every day, and even more if you're physically active. If you are exercising to lose weight (as well as trying to reduce BG levels), the following table shows calories burnt off by doing different activities for 10 minutes according to how much you weigh (in pounds – lbs):

FACT: Having an active lifestyle reduces your risk of developing Type 2 diabetes but you may still develop insulin resistance syndrome – a group of associated conditions including coronary heart disease; high blood pressure; high levels of blood fats such as cholesterol; high levels of chemicals that prevent the breakdown of blood clots in the arteries and heart; and obesity.

Activity per 10 minutes	125 lbs	150lbs	175lbs	200lbs
Climbing stairs	150	175	202	229
Running (at a pace of a mile in 9 minutes)	109	131	153	174
Aerobics (high intensity)	95	115	134	153
Swimming (moderate pace)	78	90	103	116
Tennis	75	90	105	120
Weight training	66	76	87	98
Cycling at a speed of 10 miles per hour	55	64	78	82
Golf (pulling a golf cart/carrying clubs)	46	54	62	70
Hiking	45	52	60	67
Walking (at a pace of a mile in 15 minutes)	44	52	61	70
Gardening	41	49	57	65
Shopping	35	42	49	56
Standing	20	24	28	32
Bowling	12	14	16	19
Sitting (reading or watching TV)	10	12	14	16
Sleeping	10	12	14	16

Case Study

Karen Mann has been enjoying a daily morning run for three months and, by doing this, managed to reduce her insulin needs by burning off excess blood glucose. Before she started this routine Karen's morning BG was often around 8 mmol/L with an HbA1c of 7.5% (58 mmol/L). Karen makes sure she tests her BG before her run and eats a banana to boost her carbohydrate intake to avoid hypos. Her HbA1c is now 6% (42 mmol/L).

Although exercise burns glucose, your BG can actually INCREASE after exercise. You may find that your BG is high after exercise because:

- Adrenaline released by the liver when you exercise increases BG levels, but if you have some insulin on board this available glucose will be used during the exercise.

- You have eaten too much carbohydrate to avoid a hypo because you thought it would be burned off during exercise. You may not need extra food if your BG levels are high (above 10mmol/L but less than 16.6mmol/L), or if you exercise for 20 minutes or less.

- Your BG control is generally not good and there is not enough available insulin working when you exercise. This hyperglycaemia (high BG) can cause dangerous *ketones* (fat and protein being used as fuel instead of glucose), so check your BG is stable before exercising. If you do test positive for ketones with high BG levels and have insulin, take some (1 unit of insulin usually reduces BG by 1.5 mmol/L but ask your consultant or diabetes nurse for guidance). DO NOT EXERCISE if your BG is 16.6 mmol/L or above.

FACT: Intense exercise can cause the liver to release stored glucose, increasing BG levels rather than lowering them. This is because when intense exercise is taken, there is a seven to eightfold increase in glucose production in the body and only half of this is used by the muscles.

As you've just seen under the section about HYPERGLYCAEMIA, if the exercise you do is <u>intense</u> there must be some insulin available to deal with the stored glucose released by your liver to fuel the muscles.

FACT: Exercising when BG is 16.6mmol/L and above (300 mg/dl American measurement) is not advisable as your heart has to work hard to pump syrup-like blood around the body and exercising adds an additional strain.

FACT: Eat complex carbohydrates like bread, potatoes, pasta or rice 20 minutes before you start exercising and keep a sugary drink with you to avoid hypos when exercising.

Research shows that a lack of physical activity is closely associated with a poor quality of life. This means that you can TAKE CONTROL and increase the amount of activity you do straight away and do it regularly to make it a lifestyle change to improve your diabetes.

FACT: It's easier to make a change in your lifestyle after receiving information that relates to you and your health personally, such as being told that you have an increased risk of developing Type 2 diabetes.

ALCOHOL

Alcohol acts in several ways to reduce your BG and then later raise it again when it's been processed by the body because it:

- Stops your liver from releasing glucose.
- Blocks other hormones that raise BG when it's low.
- Increases the BG-lowering effect of insulin so it works more rapidly.

You might not think of alcohol as a cause of low BG, especially if you often have a drink and haven't noticed any problems. These three effects on BG mean that drinking alcohol can cause hypoglycaemia. This is more likely to happen if you are dieting or you don't eat very much generally, especially if you drink alcohol before bed and have a hypo the following morning. This is called *fasting hypoglycaemia.*

Certain drinks, such as vodka and gin, will lower BG, so you are more likely to have a hypo. Drinking vodka and orange juice on the other hand will increase BG because of the fruit sugar in the juice. I know this might not be what you want to hear, but the key to drinking alcohol when you have diabetes is MODERATION.

Different alcoholic drinks contain differing amounts of carbohydrate so always check the bottle label to be sure. There is a substantial difference between the carbohydrate content of regular and light beer, for example, with regular beer containing 12.8 grams per small (12.5 fluid ounce) bottle, while light beer is only 5.8 grams of carbohydrate for the same amount. White wine also varies in the same way among brands, but is typically 3.8 grams of carbohydrate for a 5 fluid ounce serving (a small glass), so you might want to opt for Chardonnay at 3.2 grams of carbohydrate over the same amount of Riesling at 5.5 carbs.

FACT: If you take insulin or sulphonylurea medication, always eat some carbohydrate if you are drinking as this helps stop BG falling too low.

ASPIRIN

Aspirin, particularly in large doses, can lower BG. This is especially the case for people with Type 2 diabetes who take BG-lowering medication containing *sulphonylureas* as the aspirin helps the tablets do their job more effectively. Doctors thought at one time that this combination could be used as a different form of treatment for Type 2, but the effects weren't always the same, so this idea was abandoned. The Department of Health has advised that every adult with diabetes should take a small 75 mg dose of aspirin daily to protect against the risk of stroke and heart disease. Some over-the-counter aspirin tablets contain four times this amount (300 mg) and if you are used to swallowing two aspirins if you have a headache, this is not only a high dose but it can also significantly lower your BG. This is because aspirin can also increase the way other blood-glucose lowering drugs work (besides *sulphonylureas*), but I've not found this to be the case with insulin.

FACT: Children should never take aspirin.

Mild hypos make you feel uncomfortable, but they're NOT dangerous. If you ignore how you're feeling and don't test your blood and eat something sweet to treat the hypo, your BG may drop even lower to become a SEVERE hypo. This can be dangerous if you are on your own and lose consciousness, or if other people don't know what action to take. Always test your BG if you feel unwell because some symptoms of low and high BG are similar and everyone with diabetes experiences different warning signs. Common signs of hypo are:

MILD HYPO SIGNS
- Sweating
- Hunger
- Rapid heart beat

MODERATE HYPO SIGNS
- Irritable/aggressive behaviour
- Muscle weakness

For both mild or moderate hypos, test your BG and if you are low, eat something sweet (2–4 glucose tablets; a glass of pure orange juice or Lucozade; a small glass of non-diet fizzy drink). Follow this up with carbohydrate such as a couple of Digestive biscuits, a slice of bread, or a banana. Wait for 15–20 minutes and test again. If you are still low, the person looking after you (your hypo partner) should get you something else to eat or have a cup of tea with sugar in.

SEVERE HYPO SIGNS
- Blurred vision
- Drowsiness
- Clumsiness/appearing to be drunk
- Confusion

- Passing out (unconsciousness)
- Losing the ability to shiver if you're cold.

If you have a severe hypo and can't swallow (as it's dangerous to feed an unconscious person in case they choke), HYPOSTOP is a sugary gel that can be smeared on your lips or gums so it's absorbed into your bloodstream quickly. If you become unconscious, you will need another person to take EMERGENCY ACTION by mixing and injecting GLUCAGEN from a HYPO KIT. You will also need to have a sugary drink when you come round. If you DON'T come round, someone should dial 999.

NIGHT-TIME HYPOS

People who take insulin to treat their diabetes fear night-time hypos (*nocturnal hypoglycaemia*) when they are asleep and not able to monitor their BG every five hours or so as they would when they are awake. Many people also fear that they might have a hypo in their sleep and not wake up. This can also be a big worry for your partner and your family, and for parents of children with Type 1 diabetes. Whilst there is more likelihood that a hypo won't be detected as quickly during sleep, your brain will let you know that it needs glucose:

- You'll be woken up with symptoms of feeling shaky and sweaty, restless and irritable.
- If applicable, restlessness in bed will disturb your partner's sleep and they will wake you up so you can treat your hypo with glucose.
- Even if your hypo is severe, your body has a mechanism to release stored glucose from the liver when BG levels fall,

and this happens even when you remain asleep. You will wake up with a bad headache and feel generally unwell (similar to hangover symptoms). Because of this 'auto-correction' of BG by the body in response to a hypo, high BG levels then follow. Regularly waking and feeling like this and finding your BG is high may indicate that your BG is falling very low in the night while you sleep. I know it's a pain, but try to test your BG at three a.m. every now and again to make sure this isn't happening. If you are going low in the night, speak to your diabetes consultant or diabetes nurse for advice on altering your insulin dosages to prevent this.

FACT: If you become unconscious from hypoglycaemia you may clench your teeth. It is important that your hypo partner doesn't try to feed you anything to eat or drink when you're unconscious as you may choke.

HYPOGLYCAEMIC UNAWARENESS

Sometimes there are no symptoms of hypo. This can happen when you've had diabetes for many years and is associated with nerve damage. It can also happen if you have to take heart or blood pressure medication, where your hypo symptoms will be less obvious to you. The danger of hypoglycaemic unawareness is that you may not recognise a hypo during your sleep, so you fail to wake up from it and fall into unconsciousness, or if you drive and have no warning when your BG is dropping low. This means you have to test your BG frequently throughout the day and during the night to detect low BG results.

I have hypo unawareness and it has caused problems over the years until I began using a Continuous Glucose Monitoring (CGM) system with my insulin pump eight years ago. CGM is a sensor inserted under the skin and changed every six days to provide continual updates on BG levels every ten minutes through an insulin pump display screen. In this way I'm able to take action when the pump notifies me that my BG is dropping down low, and I can avoid a bad (severe) hypo.

FACT: If you have frequent and unpredictable hypoglycaemia with no warning signs you are a good candidate for insulin pump therapy and CGM funded by the NHS to help you manage your diabetes much better. Speak to your diabetes consultant or GP to find out more.

Having a hypo makes you feel very disorientated as your brain adjusts to having suffered low BG levels and a lack of glucose for fuel. Because of this it is a VERY good idea to have someone you trust, who understands diabetes, and someone who is around you and can help you during these situations Everyone has different experiences of what it's like to have VERY LOW BG and, although other people can see that you are not behaving normally, actually explaining what it's like is very difficult because you literally can't think straight. You may never experience the effects of a very low BG (mine were due to not having hypo warning signs before I used the glucose sensor to be able to realise I was going very low, so I reached the stage that I couldn't help myself) but if you do have very low BG levels, and so you can explain what it's like to health professionals and people close to you,

I've tried to describe below how it feels.

I've only become unconscious once since using the glucose sensor, and this is my experience in the half-an-hour following coming out of severe hypoglycaemia and unconsciousness (meaning a BG of less than 2 mmol/L or 36 mg/dl American measurement) where *Glucagen* has been injected by another person to bring me round:

- After initial sweating and feeling very hot, very low BG levels lead to a dramatic drop in body temperature (*hypothermia*) where I'm unable to get warm.

- I am left with lasting muscle weakness and confusion for several hours after coming round from unconsciousness due to my body being deprived of glucose for fuel.

- I have a very bad headache for the rest of the day and sometimes the following day as well.

- I am EXTREMELY hungry (because the body needs to replace stores of glucose in the liver) and will eat a large amount of food, not counting carbohydrates as I'm confused, and ending up with a very high BG.

- In response to low BG, my liver also releases stored glucose (a process called *counter-regulation*) and my BG then shoots up and becomes very high. This rapid increase in BG is very difficult to manage and my BG remains high for the rest of the day, despite trying to reduce it with insulin. At the same time, I also feel VERY sick because of high BG levels.

- While I'm unconscious I experience fitting (like epileptic fits) because my brain is starved of glucose and this causes brain cells to die off. Because of this, once I recover I have a complete loss of memory of events before the severe hypo.

- As I recover I'm very emotional and keep thanking the person who injected the Glucagen to get me out of the hypo situation.

FACT: As long as you have warning signs and act quickly, treat your hypo as soon as you realise it's happening so you won't become unconscious or need the help of other people.

How often should I test my BG?

This is something that you may find confusing or an unpleasant task you'd rather avoid. When you are first diagnosed with diabetes you will be asked to test your BG more frequently than when it's stabilised. If you have Type 1 diabetes or you have Type 2 and you take insulin it's advisable to test BG before meals, before driving and before bed. This is because insulin adjustments can be made according to each meal, i.e., if you often have a BG of 13 mmol/L and normally have a set dose of insulin for your evening meal, you can take a correction dosage of a couple more units to deal with the glucose you already have in your blood as well as the meal you will eat. On some evenings you may eat a more or less carbohydrate-rich meal, so the insulin you take could be too little or too much to keep BG in check.

FACT: Write the carbohydrate values of your favourite foods in a notebook so you can quickly calculate your insulin needs.

Insulin working times are also extremely important here because if your insulin works for less time than you need to cover what you've eaten, or if you have a slow rate of digestion and your insulin works too early for your needs, you will have hyperglycaemia as a result. At the other end of the scale, as we've seen, there are people with diabetes who have frequent and unpredictable hypos with little or no warning.

If this is the case, more BG tests have to be carried out to give you the confidence to be independent and in control of your condition. If you forget to test your blood occasionally throughout the day (or night) it's not something to worry about. By getting into a regular routine, as with brushing your teeth or when you first began to give yourself insulin, you will be on the right track to keeping your BG under control.

Case Study

Paul Maxwell was taking a BG-lowering medication (sulphonylurea) that had a peak working time 2-4 hours after taking it. Because Paul ate his evening meal at 8 p.m. and then went to bed a couple of hours later, he found he was having hypos while he was asleep. He had been advised that he only needed to test his BG three times a week because he had Type 2 diabetes, but Paul began to test before bed every night. He found that his BG was often only 4–4.5 mmol/L and reported this to his GP. With some adjustments to his evening carbohydrate count and his sulphonylurea dosage, Paul was able to retire to bed without the worry of having night-time hypos.

FACT: You should always test you BG before you go to sleep.

If you try to tighten your BG control, for example, if you are pregnant and keeping your diabetes as well-controlled as possible for the developing baby, you may have more hypos because there is less available glucose before you go too low. If you do make changes by increasing your insulin and you feel unwell it is important to test BG to make sure you're not having a hypo.

Now I've had Type 1 for 40 years I find that I don't always feel the same when I have low BG (not the usual symptoms as I don't have normal warning signs). Sometimes I feel really tired during the day or I get a bad headache – symptoms I've realised may be due to low BG rather than just normal life. I always test as it can be a hypo (despite what the glucose sensor tells me) and I can then take action to raise BG levels if needed.

If you have Type 2 diabetes that's treated by tablets, diet and exercise you may be advised to check your BG levels before breakfast and dinner, but if your HbA1c level is in the good range you may only need to test two to three times a week. If you take sulphonylurea medication which can cause hypoglycaemia, you will be advised to test BG several times a day. In the USA and in other countries the thinking is that frequent testing for people with Type 2 diabetes does very little to improve BG control, especially as taking tablets allows no flexibility in controlling BG in the same way taking insulin does. This is because, without being able to take additional insulin when you have a high BG level there is little you can do to lower it, other than exercise.

FACT: Always wash your hands before testing your BG as it can make a big difference to the result.

Doing repeated BG tests, especially if you have just been diagnosed with Type 1 and your consultant is trying to stabilise your insulin treatment, can make your fingers very sore. There are alternative sites for getting a blood sample other than the fingertips. The good news is that this allows your fingers to have a rest from being pricked numerous times a day. The bad news is, getting blood from sites like the upper arm, forearm, thigh or calf may not give an accurate reading because the glucose level in these parts of the body is 20–30 minutes older than in the fingertips. The fingertips and palm provide the most up-to-date BG readings. Because of this lag in current BG levels alternative sites other than the fingertips should NOT be used for blood testing if:

- You DON'T get many or any hypo warning signs (*hypoglycaemic unawareness*).
- If you are feeling low and need to know HOW low.
- You are ILL and your BG levels are running higher from infection.
- You are just about to DRIVE a vehicle.

Case Study

Kim Davies was 22 and had just been diagnosed with Type 1 diabetes. She was having difficulty getting her insulin dosages stable and her diabetes nurse advised that she should test her BG 8–10 times a day. Her fingertips were taking a battering but she persevered because she knew this would not be a long-term situation and because her BG tended to drop very quickly. After three weeks, Kim was able to test in alternative sites and reduce the number of tests to four per day.

Lifestyle changes

Case Study

Chris Jenkins was 54 and weighed 20 stone when he was told he had Type 2 diabetes. He told his doctor that eating and drinking were his only hobbies and because he enjoyed food, he wondered what was the point of making lifestyle changes to include diet and exercise. Chris saw his diabetes consultant for the first time and he agreed that Chris's diabetes was completely lifestyle-related. He added that Chris could improve his condition markedly if he steadily lost weight and did regular fat-burning exercise like cycling. Chris's family wanted him to be well and they encouraged him to follow this advice. He cut out cake, biscuits, chips and crisps from his diet and took up cycling for 5 miles three times a week with his daughter. At Chris's next diabetes clinic appointment, he was happy to be told that his diabetes was now borderline and that he could actually say goodbye to his Type 2 if he made his lifestyle changes permanent. Chris felt so much better that he did exactly that. He no longer takes Metformin.

FACT: 1 in 10 adults now risk developing Type 2 diabetes by the year 2035

FACT: Health problems related to poor diet, drinking and smoking are currently costing the NHS 11 billion pounds each year.

The key message concerning many cases of Type 2 diabetes is that YOU CAN DO SOMETHING ABOUT IT. I will be covering REVERSING Type 2 diabetes later, but it is possible to improve your BG levels enormously just by making a few small changes.

STARCHES AND SUGARS

As you have seen in the last chapter, eating any sort of carbohydrate will increase your BG, but there are different forms of carbohydrate. Potatoes, pasta and bread contain starch – GOOD carbohydrates. Sweets, cakes and biscuits are BAD carbohydrates that will raise your BG quickly and provide little nutritional value because they contain glucose or sugar. Modern diets now contain far too many bad carbohydrates and this is the reason for the sharp rise in people developing Type 2 diabetes in recent years.

By monitoring your BG and testing your urine for glucose you will be able to see exactly how eating good and bad carbohydrates makes you blood glucose level rise. You may be confused about which foods contain sugar, and there are some unexpected ones that can catch you out, like tomato sauce. Low fat foods can often fool us into thinking we're being healthy and making good choices, but by removing fat from the recipe, manufacturers often increase the amount of sugars they add to make to food taste nice.

Always READ FOOD LABELS to check exactly – if glucose syrup or sugar is the first thing on the list you can be sure that food is not for you. I once made the mistake of buying a carton of cranberry juice, thinking that is would be OK to drink as cranberries are bitter. It didn't taste particularly sweet, but my BG shot up to somewhere in the twenties afterwards. I tested a drop of cranberry juice on a BG monitoring stick (not designed for this purpose, but it worked). The reading said HI. It wasn't just being friendly – this meant the reading was so high that the meter couldn't read the glucose content. The cranberry drink was packed with sugar; like drinking flavoured glucose in juice form. I now always buy unsweetened, meaning no additional sugar has been added, but that natural sugars are still present.

If foods are marked LOW SUGAR it means they contain no more than 5% sugar per 100 grams/100 mls of food or drink. Foods marked HIGH SUGAR have 15 grams of sugar per 100 grams/100 mls, so avoid these for the sake of your BG.

CARBOHYDRATES

Being aware of how much carbohydrate there is in certain foods can help you match your diabetes medication and exercise to the food you eat. The trouble is, some carbohydrates raise BG more than others – ALL CARBOHYDRATES ARE NOT THE SAME. You may have heard of *glycaemic index* (GI) diets based on foods that raise BG the least. This is decided by how quickly your body absorbs the carbohydrate in food and converts it to glucose for fuel. The good news is that, by making a few simple substitutions in your diet, you can start eating low GI foods that raise your BG much less than high GI foods, helping you have a stable BG with fewer ups and downs. But sometimes, it's not that simple because:

- The GI of some foods may be different when eaten alone compared with if they're eaten as part of a meal.
- If you are eating, for example, a cheese sandwich, the protein and fat in the cheese can increase the GI value of the meal.
- Foods that are processed may have a different GI value to the unprocessed version.

- Although chocolate is a low GI food because it takes time to increase your BG, it has a lot of calories from fat, so it can't help you lose weight.

FACT: Don't eat chocolate to treat a hypo as it takes a long time to raise BG levels.

For these reasons the low GI diet, which seems a brilliant idea because it helps keep BG levels under control, hasn't become part of the diabetes management generally because it can be complicated. There are books you can buy on this subject that list the GI value of every food so you can make choices to suit you. A few changes you can make in your diet that will make a big difference to your glucose levels are:

- Swap white or wholemeal bread that are high GI foods for whole grain bread which contains slow-release carbohydrate.
- Eat porridge oats instead of other corn or wheat-based cereals as oats raise your BG slowly and have the effect of reducing cholesterol.
- Include biscuits that contain dried fruits or grains in your diet.
- Swap high fat, high sugar cakes for healthy options made with whole grains and fruits (this means something like a Nutrigrain bar, not an apple turnover!)
- Chose fruit that is raw or under-ripe as this contains less fruit sugar than over-ripe fruit.

- Eat a piece of fruit (not bananas, pineapple, mango, guava, or passion fruit, which contain a lot of carbohydrate) rather than drinking a glass of fruit juice.
- Swap older potatoes and instant mash for boiled new potatoes – the older the potato, the more carbohydrate it contains.
- Eat rice or pasta instead of potatoes. Long-grain rice has more carbohydrate than Basmati rice so read the labels and compare values before buying.
- Chose peas or beans (not baked beans in a tin with tomato sauce) as they are full of slow-release carbohydrates.

Because lower GI foods can make such a difference to your BG control, you will need to check your BG more often if you decide to start a low GI diet to reduce your BG. Make sure you tell your diabetes nurse or your Practice Nurse before you begin as she can help you manage your diabetes while you are making these changes. There is a lot of information to take in and consider with low GI diets, so you may decide it's not for you. Your diabetes diet, on the other hand, needs to have a certain amount of carbohydrate (low GI or not) for your insulin or BG medication to work on.

The carbohydrate content of common foods is shown below:

Food	Carb in grams
1 cup of cooked pasta or rice	45 grams
1 English muffin	30 grams
1 medium potato	30 grams
I cup of sweetcorn or peas	30 grams
Half a cup of cooked vegetables (carrots/broccoli/green beans)	15 grams
I slice of bread	15 grams
1 small piece of fruit (apple/satsuma/nectarine)	15 grams
17 grapes or 12 cherries	15 grams
Half a cup of vanilla ice cream	15 grams
2 small biscuits	15 grams
1 cup of milk	12 grams
1 six-ounce pot of unsweetened yoghurt	12 grams

Different foods with the same amount of carbohydrate raise BG in the same way, so a serving of two medium potatoes has the same carbohydrate content as one cup of vanilla ice cream – 60 grams.

FACT: In a diabetic diet, one serving of carbohydrate is measured as 15 grams.

FACT: It is the AMONT of carbohydrate that is important, not the TYPE.

You may think that choosing a sugar-free version of a food is better for you, but beware – low-sugar foods can still be HIGH IN CARBOHYDRATES. For example, a sugar-free apple pie is not made with sugar, but the fruit sugar in the apples and the carbohydrate in the flour that makes the pastry mean it will increase your BG if you eat it. When your diabetes is first diagnosed you may be advised to eat a certain amount of carbohydrate every day to balance your diabetes medication. You don't have to eat the same thing at each meal every day – as long as the carbohydrate value is the same as you've been advised, you can have the meal of your choice. It can be easy to eat more than you planned because of portion sizes. ALWAYS read food labels so you can see exactly what carbohydrate, fat and calories you are eating.

Depending on whether you are male or female you will be advised how much carbohydrate you need every day. WOMEN need 30–60 grams of carbohydrate for their main meals and 15–30 grams for snacks. MEN need 45–75 grams of carbohydrate for their main meals and 15–30 grams for snacks. Weight loss diets will contain fewer carbohydrate portions and you will be advised how to make these changes by your GP and/or diabetes team. To prevent low and high swings in BG with your carbohydrate diet:

- Don't miss meals.
- Space your meals regularly throughout the day.
- Eat balanced meals – your carbohydrate portions, lean protein and healthy fat.

You can find out the carbohydrate content of any food online at: **http://www.eatright.org/cps/rde/xchg/ada/hs.xsl/nutrition_13961 _ENU_HTML.htm**

GOOD FATS AND BAD FATS

Case Study

Julie Morris was 40, had Type 2 diabetes and ate a high fat diet. She found losing weight very difficult and her BG levels were usually high when she tested them. Julie's doctor warned her that heart disease is very common in people with

Type 2, but she said her parents and grandparents had always eaten fatty meat, butter, cheese and cream so she also did so without realising that these foods had an effect on her diabetes.

There are many types of fat. Some, like olive oil, are good for the body whilst others are bad, increasing *insulin resistance* (meaning that it cannot work properly) and levels of *cholesterol* (blood fats). ALL fats contain a high amount of calories and eating them often can mean it's hard to lose weight. The table below shows the different types of good and bad fats:

Good fats (monsaturated)	Medium fats (Polyunsaturated)	Bad fats (Saturated fats)
Rapeseed oil Olive oil (including butter substitutes) Butter substitutes made from vegetable oils (labelled high in monosaturates)	Sunflower oil Corn oil Soya oil Low-fat spreads (labelled high in polyunsaturates)	Butter Lard Block cooking fats Ghee butter and solid oils Hard margarine Fats found in pies, pastry, sausages, cakes, biscuits and full-fat cheeses

FACT: Where fat is concerned, if you generally eat low fat, low sugar foods your BG levels will be better controlled than if you often eat many high fat foods – such as pies, cakes, crisps, chips, and biscuits.

As well as checking food labels for sugar and glucose it is also wise to check the fat content before you buy. This does depend on how often you eat it and, of course, how much you eat – eating the occasional plate of cheese and biscuits is obviously not the same as a daily sausage roll or cake. Foods that are labelled LOW in fat must contain less than 3 grams of fat per 100 grams or 100 mls. REDUCED FAT foods mean they contain 25% less fat that a full-fat version but, if it's something like cheese, it is still generally high in fat. This also goes for any light version of a full fat product.

FACT: Insulin helps the body to lay down fat stores by converting glucose and other nutrients into fatty acids.

FRUIT & VEG

It's a well-known fact that eating fruit and vegetables is a good thing and we are often reminded to eat 5 portions a day to help us get valuable vitamins and minerals. People with diabetes are often short of B vitamins, necessary for a healthy nervous system; zinc, needed for growth; and vitamin D to help maintain (amongst other things) a healthy immune system. Vitamin D may be short if you don't go outside much because you are working, disabled or elderly, so check with your doctor. So, HOW MUCH is a portion of fruit or veg?

ONE portion of our five a day is:

- One piece of fruit – for example, an apple, banana or orange.
- Two smaller fruits such as plums or satsumas.
- Three tablespoons of tinned fruit in natural fruit juice (DON'T eat fruit in syrup).
- One dessert-sized bowl of salad.
- Two tomatoes.
- Three tablespoons of cooked vegetables.

FACT: Avoid buying fruit or vegetates that are unwrapped, don't need peeling, and are exposed to street traffic as they contain toxic heavy metals such as lead, aluminium, cadmium, mercury and arsenic from pollution.

Vitamins – where they can be found and how they are used by the body

- Vitamin A is found in liver, milk, carrots and green vegetables and it is needed for healthy bones and skin.
- Vitamin B1 (also known as *thiamine*) is found in meat and whole-grain cereals and is necessary for the body to convert carbohydrates into energy.
- Vitamin B2 (also known as *riboflavin*) is found in milk, cheese, fish and green vegetables and is needed for the correct metabolism (use) of food.
- Vitamin B3 (also known as *niacin*) is necessary for memory (this can improve with 140 milligrams of B3 supplement) and healthy cardiovascular function. Niacin is found in fish, lean meat and nuts and is essential for the release of energy in the body.

- Vitamin B5 (also known as pantothenic acid) is needed to break down protein, fats and carbohydrate for energy and for re-building tissues, muscles and organs. It is found in avocados, broccoli, meat, porridge, tomatoes, and wholegrains.
- Vitamin B6 (also known as pyridoxine) can be found in liver, yeast, Marmite, and brown bread. It is essential for growth.
- Vitamin B12 is found in meat and Marmite and is needed for a healthy nervous system and red blood cells.
- Folic acid (also known as Vitamin B9) is found in green leafy vegetables, potatoes, wholegrain bread and breakfast cereals with added vitamins. It is essential during pregnancy for the formation (and generally for maintenance) of a healthy nervous system and red blood cells.
- Vitamin C is found in fruit and potatoes and is needed for the maintenance of body tissues.
- Vitamin D is found in milk, cheese, yoghurt and sunlight. It is necessary for strong bones and teeth together with calcium.
- Vitamin E is found in wheat germ, wholegrain cereals and vegetable oils and is needed for maintenance of body cells.
- Vitamin K is produced by the bacteria that live in your intestines and can also be found in leafy green vegetables. It is essential for blood to clot when there is a wound.

FACT: If you have Type 2 diabetes and have been prescribed Orlistat (also known as Xenical) to treat obesity, you may be deficient in fat-soluble vitamins as a result. Orlistat works by stopping around a third of the fat you eat from being digested, so this reduces absorption of some fat soluble vitamin supple-

ments, particularly vitamins A and E. Orlistat should not be taken with Acarbose diabetes medication.

Some vitamins are needed on a daily basis because they are water-soluble and are washed out of the body in the urine, such as the vitamin B group (B1, B2, B3, B5, B6 and B12), and Vitamin C. Vitamins A, D, E and K are stored in fat globules in the bloodstream, small intestine and body tissues so we never run out. Because these vitamins are stored in the body we can have too much (a condition called *hypervitaminosis*), and this can actually cause us harm if we take large doses of vitamin supplements.

People with Type 1 diabetes and coeliac disease (an intolerance to the gluten that's added to bread) can have a vitamin D deficiency associated with this condition and may need to take supplements. ALWAYS seek advice from your doctor or dietician about taking vitamin and mineral supplements as you may need specific amounts.

Minerals – why we need them and where they can be found

Some minerals, such as calcium, are needed by the body as 'building blocks' for repair and renewal. Others, like sodium and potassium, are needed for correct nerve and muscle function and are known as *electrolytes*. This very important balance is upset when there is ketoacidosis, as the body becomes more acidic and, in severe cases, this is a medical emergency needing hospitalisation to have the body's chemical balance restored. The main role minerals have in the body is to help enzymes turn one substance into another, such as the breakdown of proteins to make new body cells. Without essential minerals, this process wouldn't happen.

FACT: All minerals are toxic to the body in large amounts. Some minerals have different variations, like chromium, and one variety may be toxic while another is essential to us. Some minerals reduce the action of other minerals in the body, such as iron, which can cause zinc deficiency because iron blocks it from working.

- Calcium, phosphorus and magnesium can be found in milk, yoghurt and cheese. These are needed for strong bones and teeth and adults should get 1,000 milligrams per day. Growing teenagers, pregnant women, and older people need 1,5000 milligrams every day. Calcium works with vitamin D to be used by the body.

FACT: BG-lowering medication can cause magnesium deficiency, ketoacidosis and irregular heart rhythm (cardiac arrhythmia) and you may need to take magnesium supplements.

- Magnesium helps convert food into energy and is important for bone health. It can be found in green leafy vegetables like spinach, nuts, brown rice, bread (especially wholegrain), fish, meat and dairy foods. Magnesium deficiency is quite common.
- Potassium is vital for the healthy function of body cells, tissues and organs and helps control water balance and

blood acidity level in the body. It is found in bananas, avocados, spinach, lentils and all fruits and vegetables.

- Selenium is important for brain function and a healthy immune system. It is also necessary for fertility in men and women. The richest source of selenium is brazil nuts (although these are also high in cholesterol), seafood and organ meats such as liver and kidney.

- Zinc helps achieve a healthy immune system and is important for cell division, to prevent cancer, to maintain healthy hormone levels ESPECIALLY insulin sensitivity, and good energy levels. Zinc is found in walnuts, Marmite, oysters, wheat germ, beef and veal. Zinc stops iron, manganese and copper from being absorbed by the body.

- Manganese can be found in many fruits and vegetables, such as raspberries, strawberries, pineapple, garlic, grapes, green beans, bananas, and in rice, nuts and oats. It is needed to maintain a healthy bone structure and brain and nervous system function, and for creating essential enzymes for building bones.

- Iron can be found in meat, dark green leafy vegetables like spinach, wholemeal bred, nuts and beans and is needed for the formation of red blood cells. Iron is needed to make the haemoglobin that caries oxygen in the blood (and is the substance that glucose sticks to, measured in a haemoglobin A1c test): ⅔ of the iron in the body makes up our haemoglobin. Women who are menstruating can become iron-deficient and anaemic, requiring iron supplements. Because iron is stored in the body tissues, a build-up of iron over time can lead to diabetes, arthritis and heart abnormalities.

- Sodium is found in salt and you only need a small amount (220 milligrams) daily. The body uses sodium to regulate the amount of water it stores. Most people eat far too much sodium in their diet, with worsened high blood pressure as a result. Sodium is added to food when it is manufactured, so cut out any additional salt added to cooking and foods like crisps, breakfast cereals, sauces and processed meats.

- Copper is needed by the body to make red blood cells and to keep nerve cells and the immune system healthy. Deficiency is rare because it is found in drinking water as it passes through copper pipes. Copper stops zinc and manganese from working.

- Chromium is found in meat, whole grains, fruit, vegetables and spices. Chromium is only needed in very small quantities by the body to reduce blood pressure, turning glucose into energy and helping insulin to work. 100 milligrams a day is recommended for good BG balance (in Type 2 diabetes).

- Iodine deficiency is extremely rare as it is added to salt (iodised salt). It is necessary for the correct functioning of the thyroid gland in the neck and the production of thyroid hormones which help the body metabolise (use) food. Apart from iodised salt, iodine is found in milk, yoghurt, cheese, seafood, mushrooms, meat and eggs.

Deficiency symptoms you many recognise

The amount of vitamins you need depends on your general health. Ideally, your intake of vitamins should be a dosage to give you the best possible health with diabetes and to prevent any symptoms of deficiency. This level can only be measured by blood tests, but you may need 50–100 times the recommended daily allowance (RDA). The RDA for vitamins and minerals varies from country to country and some essential nutrients don't have a recommended daily allowance. The RDA is the MINIMUM amount required for health: it may not be possible to gain everything you need from your diet because of various factors such as how food is grown, where it's stored, how old it is, whether it has been in direct sunlight, and how efficient your body is at processing it.

FACT: Even if we all ate the recommended daily allowance of vitamins and minerals some people would still have symptoms of deficiencies because we all have different needs.

It is natural to worry that you could be having TOO MUCH of a certain vitamin and that it could cause damage because stories in the press highlight these issues. It is claimed that vitamin A is toxic and harmful during pregnancy; that large doses of vitamin C can cause kidney stones; and that B6 in excess is dangerous for the nervous system. Vitamin A comes in animal form (retinol) which is stored in the body and vegetable form (beta-carotene), found in carrots and converted into retinol if the body needs it. Eating lots of carrots can cause yellowing of the skin because excessive beta-carotene is stored there, but it is not toxic to the body. A variety of synthetic vitamin A, (sold as *Roaccutane*), has been shown to cause toxic effects and birth defects because the vitamin A content is very high and the pregnant women involved had taken 25,000–500,000 international units a day.

Vitamin C is water soluble and if the body can't use it, any excess is excreted in the urine. There are no associations between vitamin C and kidney stones and the only adverse effect of taking very large dosages (above 3,000 milligrams per day) is that it has a laxative effect. Vitamin B6 (as with all B-vitamins) is water soluble and any excess is excreted in the urine. There has been a case of a woman who increased her daily dose of B6 from 50 to 200 milligrams over a two-year period and she developed some muscle weakness and pain that was diagnosed as nerve damage. Research studies where people took between 2,000 to 5,000 milligrams of B6 per day showed improvements in nerve function, so it may have been a case that the woman who had adverse effects had other underlying health problems causing her symptoms.

FACT: It is unlikely that you would have any symptoms of vitamin overdose from taking a daily multivitamin supplement tablet.

FACT: Supplements contain larger amounts of some vitamins that are less expensive to produce, like vitamin C. They may only contain small amounts of the vitamins or minerals you need, so always ask advice before buying them from a health food shop.

Below you will find the symptoms of deficiency for each vitamin and mineral:

VITAMIN A

Mouth ulcers; poor night vision; acne; frequent colds or infections; dry, flaky skin; dandruff; thrush or cystitis (a burning sensation when passing urine); diarrhoea.

VITAMIN D

Rheumatism or arthritis; back ache; tooth decay; hair loss; excessive sweating; muscle cramps or spasms; joint pain or stiffness; lack of energy.

VITAMIN E

Lack of sex drive; exhaustion after light exercise; easy bruising; slow wound healing (common in people with diabetes); varicose veins; loss of muscle tone; infertility.

VITAMIN C

Frequent colds; lack of energy; frequent infections; bleeding or tender gums; easy bruising; nose bleeds; slow wound healing; red pimples on the skin.

VITAMIN B1

Tender muscles; eye pains; irritability (also due to low or high BG, so make sure you check); poor concentration; 'prickly' legs and tingling hands (also a symptom of diabetic nerve damage); poor memory; stomach pains; constipation (common in people with diabetes); rapid heartbeat.

VITAMIN B2

Burning or gritty eyes; sensitivity to bright light; sore tongue; cataracts (common in people with diabetes due to high BG over time); dull or oily hair; eczema or dermatitis; split nails; cracked lips.

VITAMIN B3

Lack of energy; insomnia; headaches or migraines; poor memory; anxiety or tension; depression; irritability; bleeding or tender gums;

acne.

VITAMIN B5

Muscle tension or cramps; apathy (tiredness/no energy – also a symptom of high BG); poor concentration; burning feet (also a symptom of diabetic neuropathy) and tender heels; nausea or vomiting; exhaustion after light exercise; anxiety or tension; teeth grinding.

VITAMIN B6

Infrequent dream recall; water retention; tingling hands (also a symptom of peripheral neuropathy in people with diabetes); depression, irritability (also common in people with diabetes) or nervousness; muscle tremors or cramps; lack of energy; flaky skin.

VITAMIN B12

Poor hair condition; eczema or dermatitis; over-sensitivity to hot or cold in the mouth; irritability (also a sign of low or high BG); anxiety or tension; lack of energy (also a symptom of high BG); constipation (common in people with diabetes); tender sore muscles; pale skin.

FOLIC ACID (Also known as vitamin B9)

Eczema; cracked lips; prematurely greying hair; anxiety or tension; poor memory; lack of energy (also a sign of high BG); depression (common in people with diabetes); poor appetite; stomach pains.

CALCIUM

Muscle cramps or tremors; insomnia or nervousness; joint pain or arthritis; tooth decay; high blood pressure.

MAGNESIUM

Muscle tremors or spasms; muscle weakness; insomnia or nervousness; high blood pressure; irregular heartbeat; constipation; fits or convulsion (not the same as fits that can occur if BG is very low); hyperactivity; depression (common in people with diabetes).

IRON

Pale skin; sore tongue; tiredness/listlessness (also a sign of high BG); loss of appetite or nausea; heavy periods or blood loss.

ZINC

Poor sense of taste or smell; white marks on more than two fingernails; frequent infections; stretch marks; acne or greasy skin; low fertility (also a sign of high BG over time); pale skin; tendency to depression (common in people with diabetes); poor appetite.

MANGANESE

Muscle twitches; childhood growing pains; dizziness and poor sense of balance (not to be confused with balance problems associated with peripheral nerve damage in diabetes); fits or convulsions (also a symptom of very low BG); sore knees,

SELENIUM

Family history of cancer; signs of premature ageing (although having diabetes ages body cells more quickly due to abnormal metabolism); cataracts (common in diabetes due to high BG levels over time); high blood pressure; frequent infections.

CHROMIUM

Excessive sweating or cold sweats; dizziness or irritability after 6 hours without food (both a sign of low BG, so make sure you test your blood); cold hands (also a sign of damage to blood vessels in diabetes); need for excessive amounts of sleep or drowsiness during the day; excessive thirst (also a main symptom of diabetes due to high BG levels).

Controlling your weight

By making some changes in the amount of exercise you take and what you eat at every meal you can really make a difference to your weight. It stands to reason that replacing a chocolate bar with a banana or apple could help you reduce your daily calories. I remember being told this by my sports teacher at school, so it's not a new idea. Basically, a woman needs 2,000 calories a day and a man needs 2,500 so the body can function. If you eat more calories than you need (including those you burn off with exercise) you will put on weight. Calorie counting is an art in itself and, if you want to count everything you eat there are books available that list the calories in every kind of food you can buy. A quick guide below shows how you can make a difference to your weight and your BG by cutting out a few 100 calorie snacks each day.

Each of these is 100 calories:
3 chocolate fingers; or 2 custard creams; or 2 Jaffa cakes; or 1½ plain digestive biscuits.

2 tablespoons of double cream; or 1oz of full-fat cheese; or ½ an ounce of butter.

1 small roast potato; or 1 tablespoon of cooking oil; or ½ an ounce of sunflower spread.

7 teaspoons of jam; or 6 teaspoons of tomato sauce; or 2 tablespoons of salad cream.

5 teaspoons of sugar; or 4 barley sugars; or 1 ounce of toffee; or 1 tube f Polo mints.

½ a doughnut; or ½ a hot cross bun; or one fondant fancy.

1 small packet of crisps or ½ an ounce of salted peanuts.

2 small Yorkshire puddings; or 2 cocktail sausage rolls; or ½ a mini pork pie.

2 scoops of vanilla ice cream; or 1 dessert bowl of jelly; or 1 ladle of custard.

2 glasses of unsweetened fruit juice; or 1 small white wine; or ½ pint of beer or lager.

As you can see from this list, it's all about making choices. You may eat a couple of biscuits with your coffee or tea or a packet of crisps without even thinking about it. Be AWARE of what you're eating and when and always READ THE LABELS. If a food is high in fat, like a pie, biscuit or pastry, it will contain more calories than eating a piece of fruit instead. I was advised by my diabetes consultant as a child to eat a tomato when I wanted a packet of crisps. Not much of a swap, I thought. But we do often eat just for the sake of it rather than because we are hungry or when we need to eat because BG is low.

SMOKING

Smoking is addictive so, although you know that it isn't good for your health, it is often a difficult habit to give up. By smoking when you have diabetes you are increasing your risk of having a heart attack and/or stroke and problems with a reduced blood supply to the legs, leading to amputation risk. This is because blood vessels become narrowed and furred up so there is less room for blood to reach your brain, heart, and legs.

The NHS have said that if you give up smoking your body will feel the benefit after only 20 minutes, and the longer you don't have a cigarette or tobacco, the better:

Case Study

Jim Jenkins is 50 with Type 2 diabetes. He had smoked 20-a-day for 30 years and was always short of breath. One day he developed some worrying chest pains and he went to see his GP. Jim was told that the best thing he could do for his health was to stop smoking. He enjoyed his habit but asked for his doctor's help in quitting. Jim's GP prescribed nicotine replacement patches and told him to throw away his cigarettes and lighter. Jim found quitting wasn't easy, but with the help of the patches he gradually weaned his body off nicotine so his cravings became less and less. Jim has now been a non-smoker for two years. He admits that if someone lights up around him he thinks about having a cigarette, but his lowered risk of having a heart attack stops him.

FACT: Smoking and diabetes are a deadly combination – the likelihood of having a heart attack, stroke or blood circulation problems goes up by 4 to 9%.

Time period	Benefit to your body when you stop smoking
20 minutes	After 20 minutes, your blood pressure and pulse return to normal.
8 hours	Your chances of having a heart attack start to drop.
24 hours	Your lungs start to clear of mucus and waste products.
48 hours	Nicotine is no longer found in the body and your ability to taste and smell improve.
72 hours	Your breathing is easier and your energy levels increase.
2–12 weeks	Blood circulation increases throughout your whole body.
3–9 months	Breathing problems improve as lung function increases by 5–10%.
5 years	Your risk of heart attack is now half that of a smoker.
10 years	Lung cancer risk is half that of a smoker; heart attack risk is similar to a non-smoker.

WORK AND SLEEP

The type of work you do can actually increase your chances of developing Type 2 diabetes as well as playing a role in raising BG levels. Your metabolism (the way your body uses energy) is disrupted by a lack of sleep, so if you are getting less than 7 hours per night or your sleep is often disrupted, the insulin your own body produces (if you do not have diabetes or you have Type 2) works less well to reduce BG because of a hormonal imbalance.

The continual release of the hormones *epinephrine* and *cortisol* when you can't sleep stresses the body and this prevents the immune system working as efficiently. Epinephrine and cortisol stop other hormones, such as insulin and *serotonin* (the hormone that makes us feel happy), from working properly and over time, this can lead to illnesses like depression, heart disease, hardening of the arteries, Type 2 diabetes and certain cancers.

FACT: Insulin is 25% less effective at lowering BG levels in people without diabetes who have had disrupted sleep over 3 nights. If you have Type 1 or Type 2 diabetes and sleep problems, this could be a reason you have poor BG control and a high HbA1c.

Overwhelming evidence has shown a link between a lack of sleep and the development of Type 2 diabetes. During a normal period of 7–8 hours' undisrupted sleep the body is not expecting food. If sleep is disrupted or sleeping patterns change entirely – such as when someone does shift work – there's an increase in *insulin insensitivity* (where insulin doesn't work as well and more and more is produced to reduce BG). Insulin insensitivity starts before the development of Type 2 diabetes. People who sleep during the day and work at night are often found to have insulin insensitivity because shift work causes another hormone, *melatonin*, to be released at the wrong times. Melatonin stops insulin working properly and causes higher BG levels when a person doing shift work eats something. This is not the same as Type 2 diabetes – it is the way the body reacts to sleep deprivation or shift work BEFORE Type 2 develops begins.

SEX

FACT: Unfortunately having diabetes can have a big impact on this area of your life if BG control is not good.

WOMEN

With regard to a reduced sex drive in women with diabetes, there is very little information available about this topic: most of the researchers in this area are men, and so the focus has been on erectile dysfunction as the major sexual issue in people with diabetes. A normal sex drive in women with diabetes is achievable with good BG control as high glucose levels cause dryness of the mouth and vagina, thrush infections, and can be the cause of an irregular menstrual cycle. A low or non-existent sex drive may be due to psychological issues like poor self-esteem. If you have any problems with this area of your life it is important to speak to your doctor or diabetes specialist who can refer you to a counsellor or psychologist specially trained in diabetes-related issues.

In terms of fertility, women can find it difficult to become pregnant if their HbA1c and general diabetes control is poor. If you are planning to become pregnant you should consult your GP and/or your diabetes care team as they can help you to achieve the best possible BG control to enable a healthy conception and pregnancy. Pregnancy for diabetic mothers is definitely more complicated than for mothers without the condition. Your GP, midwife and diabetes care team will be aware of this and may suggest you have your baby in one of the specialised birthing centres around the country that can provide up-to-date technology and expertise.

FACT: If the mother already has diabetes the child is 6 times more likely to develop it.

FACT: If you have Type 1 diabetes and become pregnant your insulin needs will change. If you have Type 2 diabetes you will be advised to stop taking glucose-reducing tablets and change to insulin injections while pregnant (you should be able to return to tablets after the birth). If gestational diabetes develops while you're pregnant you will be advised to reduce your carbohydrate intake and may need to take insulin while you are pregnant.

Pregnancy and Type 1 diabetes

If you have Type 1 diabetes and become pregnant your insulin needs will double or even treble. This need usually begins to fall several weeks before the birth until in the last week or fortnight you actually become hypo more often. When your baby is born your insulin needs will fall dramatically as your BG eventually returns to pre-pregnancy levels. You will be advised to eat less carbohydrates after the birth and to regularly monitor you BG levels, so insulin needs will be reduced.

If you already suffer from diabetic eye disease (*retinopathy*) and the condition is severe this may get worse while you are pregnant. This is also a possibility if you make drastic improvements to your BG control because you are pregnant. This worsening of diabetic retinopathy is ironically due to improved BG levels in blood reaching the tiny blood vessels (capillaries) in the eyes. This situation reverses when your baby is born and your eyesight becomes the same as it was before your pregnancy. Diabetic kidney damage (*nephropathy*) may also become worse during pregnancy, but this situation usually reverses after the birth.

FACT: If the mother had high BG levels and ketones during pregnancy the baby may have impaired intelligence as it becomes older.

Pregnancy and Type 2 Diabetes

Women with Type 2 diabetes are more likely to develop high blood pressure when they become pregnant. You will be advised to monitor your BG more frequently during your pregnancy. Most women with Type 2 will be able to go the full-term of 39 weeks but if you do have high blood pressure, or you had a previous difficult delivery, you may be advised to not go to full-term.

Case Study

Gloria Sanchez was 35 with Type 2 diabetes for three years before she became pregnant with her fourth child. Gloria was advised by her diabetes team to stop her glucose-reducing medication as it was not good for the baby, and her consultant started her on insulin. She soon got used to testing her BG before and after meals and adjusting her insulin accordingly. Gloria was also given nutrition education by the hospital dietician and told to reduce her daily calories, and to eat smaller meals to even out her BG levels. One week later Gloria's BG tests were within normal range most of the time and she went on to have a healthy, normal weight baby boy.

Pregnancy and gestational diabetes

Varying BG levels during pregnancy mean that tests to determine gestational diabetes in the mother are often inaccurate. This means that the condition is hard to diagnose and there is no definition of BG level to confirm that someone definitely has gestational diabetes. In a glucose tolerance test where 75 grams of glucose is given by mouth, a result after two hours that is above 7.8 mmol/L (140.4 mg/dl American measurement) but below 11.1 mmol/L (199.8 mg/dl) is generally accepted as IMPAIRED GLUCOSE TOLERANCE.

A result above 11.1 mmol/L after two hours is diagnosed as GESTATIONAL DIABETES. Although BG levels are higher, because gestational diabetes develops from the twentieth week of pregnancy there is little chance of birth defects from hyperglycaemia because the baby's development is more advanced than if the mother has high BG levels from conception.

FACT: 18% of pregnant mothers develop gestational diabetes in their 20th week.

Issues in early pregnancy

The most important factor when you have diabetes and become pregnant is to have the best possible BG levels. Miscarriages and birth defects are caused by poor diabetes control at conception and during the first five to nine weeks of the baby's development. This can be the time BEFORE a woman knows she is pregnant, meaning that BG control may not have been good. The downside of trying to tighten your BG control is that you may have more hypos because there is less glucose available if you are doing the same activities every day. This is more likely during early pregnancy but your mild hypos won't harm the baby. TEST YOUR BG throughout the day and also occasionally during the night.

Late pregnancy

During the later stages of pregnancy, larger babies are the main problem for mothers with diabetes. LARGE is defined as 4.5 kilos or 9.9 pounds or above at birth. When a non-diabetic mother has a large baby its development is in line with its size but, as we've seen, large babies born to diabetic mothers are not fully matured. If diabetes is undiagnosed and BG levels are not reduced, the risk of birth defects is high as excess glucose causes areas of the baby where fat is stored to become enlarged. The baby will generally lose this excess weight during the first year but has an increased risk of becoming obese from age six to eight years.

FACT: Having poor BG control during pregnancy can mean the baby becomes abnormally large because its pancreas is producing insulin to reduce BG and this causes a high amount of fat to be stored in its shoulders, chest, abdomen, arms and legs. Large babies are delivered early although they are not full term. Controlling your BG can prevent your child becoming obese or even developing diabetes themselves.

FACT: Taking 400 micrograms of folic acid daily from a month before you conceive to 12 weeks into your pregnancy helps your baby's spinal cord to develop normally.

MEN

Erectile dysfunction

Men with diabetes may have problems because of erectile dysfunction. Although this is something that you may not talk about, more than half of men with diabetes say they have problems with sexual function and for men over the age of 70, this increases to more than three-quarters of older men with the condition. This is not just a problem seen in men with diabetes – one in ten men WITHOUT diabetes also suffer in this way. Your diabetes MAY NOT be to blame though as there are several reasons why a man cannot get and sustain an erection:

- If you smoke, drink alcohol, and/or take illegal drugs such as cannabis.
- If you suffer an accident that affects your penis (i.e., you have scar tissue).
- If you have hormonal problems such as too little *testosterone* or too much *prolactin*.

- You have nerve damage due to surgery to your prostate gland, bowels or bladder.
- You have poor blood supply to the penis due to *peripheral vascular disease.*
- You have psychological problems such as anxiety, depression or stress.
- You have suffered spinal cord damage.

Poor BG control over many years can lead to nerve damage so a man cannot have or sustain an erection. Nerve damage happens for the following reasons:

- BG control that is not within normal limits (ideally between 5–7 mmol/L). The worse your BG control the greater the risk of nerve damage.
- The length of time you have had diabetes has an impact – the longer you've had it the more likely it is that your will have erectile problems.

Treatments

Luckily for men with diabetes, treatments are available for erectile dysfunction. Both *Viagra* and *Levitra* have been designed specifically to improve blood flow to the penis. These drugs have a 70% success rate but they do have some side-effects, such as headaches, flushing of the face and indigestion. Other effects are having a hint of colour in your vision, blurring of eyesight, and increased sensitivity to light. These problems tend to get better the longer the drugs are used. A third drug used for erectile dysfunction,

Uprima (prescribed for angina, low blood pressure and heart failure), can be dissolved under the tongue and is effective after 20 minutes. Side-effects of Uprima are nausea (feeling sick), headaches, dizziness, yawning, not being able to sleep, sweating, flushing of the skin and an altered taste sensation (some of these symptoms are similar to those of low BG).

FACT: Viagra, Levitra or Uptima SHOULD NOT be taken with nitrate drugs prescribed for chest pain as this may cause a sudden and potentially fatal drop in blood pressure.

- It is also possible for a man to inject his penis to relax the blood vessels to allow more blood to enter. This can only be done two to three times a week.
- A small pill called *Alprostadil* can be inserted via a tube into the opening of the penis after which the tube is removed. This can be used twice in 24 hours.
- Devices that fit over the penis to create pressure allow blood to enter the tissues. A rubber band is then placed around the base of the penis to retain the blood and this can be kept in place for 30 minutes. Some pain and numbness may occur.
- Penis implants can be used if none of the above alternatives appeal. This provides a permanent erection. As this may be unwanted, an inflatable device containing fluid can be implanted into the scrotum to inflate the penis when desired.

FACT: If you have diabetes you will be eligible for ANY of these remedies for erectile dysfunction on the NHS. If your GP writes 'SLS' on your prescription this will be issued free of charge.

GETTING BACK CONTROL

'I used to be on tablets but I now take insulin and I feel great!'

You will already have gathered from the case studies in other chapters that there are several treatment options available depending on the type of diabetes you have. Type 1 diabetes is treated with insulin, but it can be introduced into the body by injection, insulin pen or insulin pump. People with Type 2 diabetes may be able to control the condition with diet and exercise; diet, exercise and BG-lowering medication; or have to move from tablets to insulin if they become pregnant or if the tablets no longer control BG levels as well as they used to.

Insulin injections and insulin pens

Insulin is used to control BG levels in Type 1 diabetes where the body no longer produces it, or in Type 2 diabetes where the body no longer uses the insulin it makes properly, and tablets cannot control BG. Insulin works by moving glucose from the blood into the body tissues so it can be used for energy. Insulin also stops the liver from producing even more unnecessary glucose. Some types of insulin work very quickly and others work over many hours:

RAPID-ACTING INSULIN: (Humalog; Novolog; Apidra) is taken before meals to cover the associated BG rise. This is used with long-acting insulin and it takes 10–30 minutes to reach the bloodstream where it works for 3–5 hours.

SHORT-ACTING INSULIN: Regular (R) insulin is taken 30 minutes before a meal to cover the rise in BG. This is used with long-acting insulin and takes 30 minutes to 1 hour to reach the bloodstream, where it works for 12 hours.

INTERMEDIATE-ACTING (NPH INSULIN): covers the BG rise when rapid-acting insulin stops working. It is usually taken twice a day with rapid- or short-acting insulin, taking 1½ to 4 hours to reach the bloodstream where it works for up to 24 hours.

LONG-ACTING INSULIN: (Lantus and Levemir) is usually combined with rapid- or short-acting insulin. It reaches the bloodstream from 40 minutes to 4 hours where it works for up to 24 hours.

FACT: It's easier if you WRITE DOWN when you should take your insulin and how much.

Insulin comes in vials (small bottles) for use in syringes and insulin pumps, and pre-filled devices or cartridges to use with insulin pens. It is important to ALWAYS CHECK when you receive your prescription to make sure it is the right type and that you have been given the right things you need to take it, i.e., syringes or needles. I never used to do this and trusted the pharmacist to get it right until one day I found that a new receptionist at my GP surgery had ordered me insulin pen cartridges instead of vials of insulin. Luckily I had enough insulin in my fridge to cover me until I picked up the right prescription.

You will be taught how to draw up and inject insulin or how to use an insulin pen when you are first diagnosed with Type 1, or when your consultant decides you need insulin if you have Type 2.

FACT: You should never re-use of share needles or syringes. Put used 'sharps' in a puncture-proof container and ask your doctor or pharmacist how you can dispose of this.

Case Study

Rajesh Karamel had Type 2 diabetes and his consultant told him he needed to take insulin because his tablets weren't bringing his BG down as well as they used to. He needed both short- and long-acting insulin and had to learn how to mix the two in one syringe for injection. He was advised to always draw up the cloudy, long-acting insulin into the syringe first before the clear, short acting insulin. After Rajesh had done this a few times it became second nature to take his insulin instead of a tablet.

THE DOs AND DON'Ts OF INSULIN

- DO store insulin in the fridge – it is a protein.

- DO always check your insulin before you inject it. Regular insulin (such as Humalin R or Novoin R) should be clear and colourless like water.

- DO warm the insulin to room temperature between your hands before injecting it.

- DO shake or rotate insulin to mix it before drawing it up if you are told to do so.

- DON'T use Regular insulin if it looks cloudy, thick, coloured, or if there are bits floating in it. NPH insulin (such as Humalin N; Novolin N; or pre-mixed insulin containing NPH such as Humalin 70/30 or Novolin 70/30) SHOULD look cloudy or milky after they are mixed.

- DON'T use any kind of NPH insulin if there are bits floating in the mixture or solid white particles stuck to the bottom or sides of the bottle.

- DON'T use insulin that is past the expiry date printed on the outer packaging.

- DON'T ever mix fast- and slow- acting insulin in a syringe unless you are told to by your diabetes consultant or nurse.

INJECTION SITES

Insulin can be injected beneath the skin into the backs of your upper arms, thighs, abdomen or buttocks (it's not so easy to inject yourself here as you can't see what you're doing). Injecting insulin into MUSCLE makes it work more quickly than in fat and I only do this if I have a very high BG that I need to get down as fast as possible. Take care not to inject your insulin in the same place every time because it doesn't work as well and the area may become a fatty lump. Make sure you rotate your injection sites and, for example, use your upper arm in the morning and thigh in the evening. If you do inject in the same area, do it at least half an inch from your previous injection. NEVER inject insulin into skin where there is a scar or a mole.

FACT: You cannot take insulin by mouth because, as a protein, insulin is broken down by digestion.

Case Study

Sharon Benson had been injecting insulin for her Type 1 diabetes for 5 years although she had a severe needle phobia. Her GP suggested that she try an insulin inhaler to deliver insulin directly to her lungs so it could enter her bloodstream. It was not a treatment widely available on the NHS, but Sharon's doctor agreed this was a special case. Sharon was excited to try this new way of taking insulin and, because she had never smoked and did not have asthma, she was told it would make a real improvement to her diabetes control. When Sharon tried the insulin inhaler she found there were a few problems like a sore throat, cough and some hypos, but she stuck with it in preference to taking injections and has now been giving herself insulin this way for six months. She says that it makes her feel liberated and free.

Insulin pumps

Insulin pump therapy has been around since the 1970s and is a different way of getting insulin under the skin. This happens through a small tube (cannula) inserted inside a needle. The tube is connected to a reservoir (syringe) of insulin that fits inside the pump. This is renewed and refilled every 2-3 days (or when BG levels start to rise because the fat under the skin around the insulin infusion site – where the insulin goes in – becomes over-absorbed with insulin so it can't work properly. The pump delivers a continuous background rate of fast-acting insulin (the *basal rate*) and can be programmed to give a larger dose (*bolus*) of insulin to cover the rise in BG when you eat. For some people (and I'm one of them) an insulin pump helps achieve much better control of diabetes than with injected insulin because the dosages delivered are set according to need during the day and night.

FACT: Insulin pump therapy is also known as CSII – Continuous Subcutaneous Insulin Infusion, IPT, pump therapy, insulin infusion therapy, and intensive insulin treatment.

An insulin pump is battery driven and is about the size of a pager (three and a half inches by two inches) and has an area for the reservoir of insulin to be inserted when connected to a thin plastic tube. This *infusion set* is inserted into the fat under the skin by the pump user (this doesn't hurt). The pump can also be connected to a continuous glucose sensor which measures the glucose level in the liquid part of the blood (plasma) every 10 minutes. This is especially usefully for managing frequent and unexplained hypos (meaning that there's no reason why they happen) and for people with absent or very reduced hypo symptoms.

The pump comes in a range of colours and styles and is made by several different medical companies, so there is plenty of choice although they all do the same job of delivering insulin. Pump therapy is sometimes started as soon as a person is diagnosed with Type 1 diabetes in the UK as erratic swings in BG levels can be managed much more easily this way than with multiple daily injections (MDI) of insulin. Pump therapy is especially useful for controlling BG levels:

- When there is hypoglycaemia unawareness.
- In children.
- In women who want to conceive or who are pregnant.
- In people with brittle (difficult to manage) Type 1 diabetes.

Not surprisingly, an insulin pump is expensive if you want to buy one yourself, costing around £2,500 and £800 a year for the tubing (insulin infusion sets) and reservoirs (syringes) and batteries that go with it. For people with difficult to control Type 1 diabetes, and some people with Type 2 who are on insulin, the Department of Health will fund this treatment. If it's felt that you have a CLINICAL NEED for pump therapy because you are unable to manage your diabetes well with multiple daily insulin injections and/or you have developed some chronic complications because of this, your diabetes consultant will write a letter to your local medical funding committee (CCG – County Commissioning Group). This will put the case to show you have a clinical need for the treatment because your diabetes cannot be managed well any other way.

The real benefit of using a pump is that good control of BG levels can be achieved to prevent or manage any complications that develop through long-term high or poor BG levels. In some countries in Europe, pump therapy is automatically started as soon as a person is diagnosed with Type 1 because the cost of treating chronic diabetic complications (cataract surgery or kidney dialysis, for example) costs far more than funding this treatment.

FACT: A pump cannot just be 'plugged in' and forgotten about – the user receives intensive training about how to use this technology properly and effectively.

The user has to know exactly how to get the best out of pump therapy and must be prepared to 'intensively self-manage' their diabetes with frequent BG tests to give the right amount of insulin at the right times. As I've already mentioned, a further piece of technology that works with the pump is a glucose sensor (*Continuous Glucose Monitor*, or CGM). This is also inserted under the skin and then attached to a small transmitter that sends glucose results every ten minutes to the pump so the user is warned if they are going too high or too low. This is very useful if you no longer have warning signs of hypos, especially during the night.

FACT: Although there are several different makes of insulin pump on the market that all work in the same way, you may wonder if any make is better than anther – they are all equally good!

Case Study

Daniel Morgan was 8 years old when his mum, Kelly, first told his diabetes consultant of the difficulties she was having controlling Daniel's BG levels during the night. The consultant felt that a pump would be the answer by providing measured doses of insulin throughout the night rather than one larger injected dose that was working all at once to cause Daniel's night-time hypos and early morning high BGs as a result. Kelly was worried that Daniel would not adapt to using the pump and that it might be damaged or become disconnected with him running around in the playground with his friends at school. The consultant assured Kelly that pumps are made from the same material as crash helmets and that the infusion set is taped onto the skin of the abdomen, so was unlikely to pull out. Kelly and Daniel attended the hospital a fortnight later to be shown how to use the pump by the diabetes nurse. Daniel has now been successfully using his 'insulin box' for six months and he no longer has low and high BG swings during the night.

Case Study

Anna Chatterjee was 24 with poor BG control when she decided to try for a baby. Her consultant advised that her Type 1 diabetes would be much better managed if she used an insulin pump because her dosages could be tailored to her needs if she was prepared to do regular BG tests. Anna agreed that she wanted her baby to be as healthy as possible and began using a pump to deliver her insulin 3 months before she conceived. Her HbA1c tests remained constantly within normal rage throughout Anna's pregnancy and she had a 5½ pound baby girl without any problems. Anna's consultant agreed that because she had been able to improve her BG control so much by using an insulin pump, she should continue to use it to manage her diabetes effectively.

Advantages of insulin pump therapy over insulin injections or pens:

- An insulin dosage (bolus) can be taken just before a meal or over several hours following a meal if there is slow stomach emptying.
- Dosage adjustments of background (basal) insulin help avoid BG swings.

- A bolus of insulin can be given for an unplanned meal or snack, and meals don't have to be eaten at certain times.
- The pump can be easily disconnected to take a shower or bath.
- There is a safety feature where a maximum dose can be set to prevent insulin overdose.

Disadvantages of pump use:
- A pump is worn on the outside of the body and this shows other people you have diabetes, although it's the size of a pager and no one has ever asked me what it is that I'm wearing.
- Pumps are not waterproof so have to be taken of when bathing or swimming.
- The insulin in the reservoir can warm up so it doesn't lower BG as well in very hot weather

FACT: Using insulin pump therapy is a lifestyle change as it is an INTENSIVE INSULIN TREATMENT. This means that you have to be prepared to test your BG numerous times a day, be willing to act on the results and use technology to fine tune your diabetes self-management to be as good as it can be.

Glucose-lowering tablets

There are many glucose-lowering medications available to treat and manage Type 2 diabetes:

Medication name	When to take it	Effects
BIGUANIDES Metformin (Glucophage) Metformin liquid (Riomet) Metformin extended release (Glucophage XR, Foramet, Glumetza)	Taken twice a day with breakfast and evening meal. Usually taken once a day in the morning.	Bloating, wind, diarrhoea, upset stomach, loss of appetite in first few weeks of taking. Take with food to reduce these effects. Unlikely to cause low BG. There may be lactic acid acidosis in people with reduced kidney and liver function.
SULPHONYLUREAS Glimepiride (Amaryl) Glyburide (Diabeta, Micronase) Glipizide (Glucotrol, Glucotrol XL) Micronized Glyburide (Glynase)	Taken twice a day with meals.	These stimulate insulin production & can cause low BG, so carry glucose tablets with you. Follow your meal & exercise plan and tell your GP if you have consistently low BG. If your activity increases or your weight decreases your dose may need to be lowered.
MEGLITINIDES Repagunide (Prandin) D-Phenylalanine derivatives Nanteglinide (Starlix)	Taken once a day at same time each day.	Works quickly & stop working quickly. May cause low BG but less likely to do so than sulphonylureas.

THIAZOLIDINES Pioglitazone (TZDS) Pioglitazone (Actos)	Taken once a day at same time each day.	Swelling/fluid retention. These tablets increase the amount of glucose taken up by muscles, stop glucose over-production by the liver, but don't cause low BG. May improve blood fat levels. Increases risk of congestive heart failure in people at risk.
DPP-4 INHIBITORS Sitagiptin (Januvia) Saxaguptin (Oxglyza) Linaglyptin (Tradienta)	Take one a day at the same time each day.	Stomach discomfort, diarrhoea, stuffy nose, sore throat, upper respiratory infection. Do not cause low BG & can be taken with Metformin, a sulphonylurea or Actos.
ALPHA-GLUCOSIDASE INHIBITORS Acarbose (Precose) Miglitadol (Glyset)	Take with first bite of your meal; if not eating, don't take.	Slows absorption of carbs into bloodstream. Can initially cause wind, diarrhoea, abdominal pain. Take with meals to limit a rise in BG after meals. These do not cause low BG.

BILE ACID SEQUESTRANTS Colesevelam (Welchol)	Take once or twice a day with meals. Works with diabetes medication to lower BG. May interact with contraceptives, glyburide, levothyroxine (take thyroid medication & glyburide 4 hours before Welchol).	Constipation, headache, wind, diarrhoea, nausea, heartburn. Used to lower cholesterol. Tell your GP if you have high blood fats or stomach problems, or if you have effects from these tablets that don't go away.
COMBINATION PILLS Pioglitazone & Metformin Actoplus Met Glyburide & Metformin (Glucovance) Glipizide & Metformin (Metaglip) Sitagliptin & Metformin (Janumet) Saxagliptin & Metformin (Kombiglyze) Repaglinide & Metformin (Prandimet) Pioglitazone & Glimerpiride (Duetact)	Usually taken once a day; combines the action of each tablet.	Side effects are same as each pill and combination may cause low BG. Combination may reduce amount of pills you take.

Other information you should know

As you can see from the long list above, BG-lowering tablets do this in different ways and some of these medications can have side-effects. One of the first diabetes medications you may be given for Type 2 are any of the SULPHONYLUREAS listed. These may cause rashes and weight gain and you may also reach a point where they fail to reduce your BG, even if you increase the dose. If this happens your consultant will reduce your dose back to the level where it was working well.

METFORMIN can cause an upset stomach, although this improves if the tablets are taken with food. Other possible effects are weight loss and while you might be happy about this, it is due to nausea and diarrhoea, often accompanied by a poor appetite for food. Intestinal disturbances may also lead to poor absorption of vitamin B12 which helps keep your blood and nervous system healthy.

Some groups of people may be advised not to take Metformin, such as those with poor kidney or liver function; 0ics and pregnant and nursing mothers who will be put onto insulin. Taking Metformin with the indigestion medication, *cimetidine* can increase the amount of Metformin working in the body. You will be advised to stop taking Metformin for a couple of days if you are having surgery or an x-ray involving the injection of dye.

ACARBOSE should not be taken during pregnancy (insulin will be prescribed to you instead); if you suffer from inflammatory bowel disease (such as Crohn's disease or ulcerative colitis); or if you have reduced liver or kidney function, a hernia, or if you have previously had abdominal surgery.

Case Study

Sheila Watkins had just started seeing a new man, Frank, and her consultant had also just started her on Acarbose to treat her Type 2 diabetes. Sheila had been warned that she could experience an upset stomach and wind. A few days later Sheila met with Frank for a meal out, only to find that she had continual aromatic wind throughout the evening which completely ruined her date. Sheila was so horrified by the experience and, convinced that Frank was completely disgusted with her, Sheila phoned him to apologise and say she perfectly understood if he didn't want to see her again. To her surprise, Frank just laughed, adding that he also took Acarbose and that if she'd told him, he could have warned her about the side effects in the first few weeks!

GLITAZONES have the best effect on BG after eating because they are quickly absorbed; improve insulin resistance; and reduce the amount of insulin the body has to produce to reduce BG. These tablets take two to three months before they start working to full effect (so they are usually taken with another medication such as Metformin to reduce BG). These tablets can lead to weight gain of 1–4 kilograms over the first six months of taking them. They can also cause fluid retention in the lower legs (*oedema*) and iron deficiency (*anaemia*). Be warned that cases of improved fertility and unexpected pregnancy have been reported! These tablets should not be taken by people with poor liver or kidney function or by pregnant or breastfeeding mothers.

MEGLITINIDES are broken down by the liver so if you have poor liver function, the dose of these tablets will be reduced. If liver disease is advanced you will be advised NOT to take Meglitinides. If you have kidney impairment, any increase in the dose should be carefully monitored by your GP and diabetes consultant. These tablets sometimes cause a rash to develop, and/or a stomach upset and vomiting in the case of allergy to this medication. Pregnant and breastfeeding women, people under 18 or over 75, and people with severe liver disease should NOT take Meglitinides.

Know your enemy!

The reason for trying to get the best possible BG control is to avoid or delay the development of long-term complications. You may have heard this word a few times in connection with diabetes, especially if you have had no symptoms of Type 2 diabetes and have been living with high BG levels for a few years. Unfortunately, serious medical problems can happen whatever type of diabetes you have, and these may take up to 10 years to appear after a period of poor BG control.

FACT: You can do a lot to reduce your risk of developing these problems.

HOW DO THESE PROBLEMS START?

When BG levels are high your blood becomes thick like syrup so your heart has to work much harder to pump it around your body. The glucose in your blood sticks to the sides of blood vessels, narrowing the amount of space available for your blood to flow through. The amount of glucose that attaches to your red blood cells over three months (the life span of these cells) is measured in an HbA1c test. Glucose can also attach itself to white blood cells and other substances in the blood, so if glucose levels are higher than anything up to the normal 6% (42 mmol/L) this can change the function of cells – red blood cells are unable to hold as much oxygen, and white blood cells are not able to fight infection.

These changes in cell function start the development of complications. Another abnormal process in the body when it is trying to use glucose as fuel but there is too much glucose is that it breaks it down into harmful toxins. Body cells also shrivel up because the water balance inside and outside the cell is affected. Genetic factors may also be a cause of complications.

FACT: One in six NHS beds is currently taken up by a person with Type 1 or Type 2 diabetes and complications.

WHAT KINDS OF COMPLICATIONS ARE THERE?

There are many complications that may develop after a period of poor BG control. The first to usually develop are eye, nerve and/or kidney problems. Smaller blood vessels, such as those at the back of the eyes, become weaker and may leak or burst. Larger blood vessels that supply your heart, brain and legs are also more likely to become blocked. High amounts of glucose do not just cause problems with blood vessels. Nerves are also affect, particularly the ones in your feet. I appreciate that this subject is depressing, but the good news is...

DIABETIC COMPLICATIONS ARE NOT INEVITABLE!

KIDNEYS

Because your kidneys filter urine containing high amounts of glucose, i.e., before your diabetes is diagnosed, if your diabetes is poorly controlled, or when your BG is high because you have an infection, damage is caused. Glucose molecules are large, doing much damage to the structures that cleanse the blood as they pass through urine filtration membranes within the kidney. These become thicker and expand into the space occupied by the small blood vessels. Because diabetic kidney disease (*nephropathy*) is not painful, this damage can go on over many years undetected. After 15 years the problem may become severe and blood tests show major kidney malfunction and after 20 years, the kidneys can fail entirely. But don't panic!

FIRSTLY, glucose is only present in the urine when your BG reaches 10mmol/L or above. SECONDLY you will be asked by your GP and/or diabetes consultant to provide a urine sample at least every year. This is tested for the presence of small amounts of protein – the first stage of kidney disease. If this is found you will be prescribed medication to slow the progression of the disease. THIRDLY tightening BG control is the best way to tackle or prevent the first stage of diabetic kidney disease. I was diagnosed with this in 1994 and I was prescribed medication. I did some reading up on the subject, tightened my BG control, and when I had the next lot of tests my kidney function was shown to be normal again, so the tablets were not needed. Result! Other factors that are known to contribute to kidney damage are: high blood pressure; high blood fats such as cholesterol; genetic factors such as ethnicity; and smoking.

EYES

Having diabetes can affect your eyes in several ways, again because of higher than normal BG levels. CATARACTS happen when the lens of the eye develops opaque areas that can block vision. These develop far more often in people with diabetes of all ages than in the non-diabetic population. When a cataract is mature it is surgically removed, a plastic lens is implanted to replace your own and your sight can be as good as it always was. GLAUCOMA is a disease where there is increased pressure within the eye which may damage the optic nerve. It is a common problem in people with diabetes and if it is not checked regularly, it can cause blindness because the optic nerve is destroyed, but medical treatment can lower this pressure.

RETINOPATHY is the name for diabetic changes to the retina at the back of the eye. This is due to high BG levels over time and can cause blindness if left untreated. The first changes are seen after 10 years in both Type 1 and Type 2 diabetes. There are different types of retinopathy that are categorised by their potential to cause visual loss: *Background retinopathy* (stable but can cause problems); retinal haemorrhages and hard exudates (capillary bleeds and leaked yellow fat deposits that cause scarring); macular oedema (fluid build-up causing loss of vision); and cotton wool spots and soft exudates (decreased blood supply to the nerves and destruction of the nerves of the retina). These changes can go on to become *proliferative retinopathy* which, if untreated, causes loss of vision.

You are more likely to develop retinopathy if:

- You are of South Asian origin.
- If you have certain genetic factors as well as your diabetes.
- You have high blood pressure.
- You have a long duration of diabetes (I have non-proliferative retinopathy after 40 years).
- You smoke or drink alcohol

There is no medication you can take for retinopathy, but laser surgery has saved the vision of many people. There are some risks with this procedure: minor loss of vision due to burns to the retina, a small reduction in night-time vision and a reduction in the visual field that the treated eye can take in. Both eye and kidney disease often go hand in hand:

Case Study

Mia Villano was 34 when she developed proliferative retinopathy and nephropathy within six months of one another. She said her eyesight was like looking through a piece of gauze although she wasn't even aware of her kidney problems because there was no pain or other symptoms. Her consultant told her that eye and kidney problems are also associated with cardiovascular problems. Her complications had developed due to repeated bouts of ketoacidosis as a result of very high BG levels as a teenager.

Eye screening

There is a National Screening Programme for Diabetic Retinopathy. If you are over 11 years old with diabetes you will be offered photographic eye screening every year to check the back of your eye (the retina). You can find out more about this on the website at **www.nscretinopathy.org.uk** Screening will only pick up diabetic changes in the retina, so it doesn't detect problems like cataracts or glaucoma. In some cases, these problems will be seen during the screening process and you will be referred to the hospital eye clinic directly or to your GP for more checks.

It is VERY IMPORTANT to have your eyes screened for diabetic retinopathy because:

- Untreated diabetic retinopathy is one of the most common causes of blindness in the working-age population.
- If detected early, laser treatment is very effective at reducing sight loss from diabetic retinopathy.
- Diabetic retinopathy does not usually affect your sight until the changes to your retina are fairly advanced. By this stage laser treatment is less-able to reduce sight loss.

Screening your eyes for diabetic retinopathy means regular examinations to detect any diabetic changes that could affect your sight. These changes are known as *sight-threatening diabetic retinopathy.* Screening will decide whether you need to be followed up with treatment from the hospital eye clinic for diabetic retinopathy. If you have no diabetic changes, or if your existing retinopathy is stable, you will be asked to come back for screening a year later.

FACT: Everyone over the age of 11 with diabetes needs to have eye screening. This is the case if you take insulin OR tablets OR you use diet and exercise to manage your BG levels, and whether you see your GP OR a diabetes specialist for your diabetes care.

If you ALREADY VISIT a hospital eye clinic for another eye condition, and then you develop diabetes, the doctor you already see there will take over your eye screening. Make sure this doctor is aware that you have diabetes so they specifically check for diabetic retinopathy each year – hospital clinics tend to have visiting eye specialists with them for a year before they move to another hospital so you won't get to see the same person each time.

FACT: You will still need to visit your optician every one to two years for sight tests, glasses or contact lenses.

So, what actually happens during retinal screening?

- Your GP, hospital, local retinal screening programme or mobile unit in your area will have your details and are bound by a duty of care and confidentiality.
- You will be invited to attend a screening appointment by letter in the post. The screening may be at your GP's surgery, your opticians, at the local hospital, or another convenient local venue to you if it is a mobile screening unit.
- The procedure will be explained when you arrive and you can ask any questions you have about the screening.
- They will take a record of your details and your level of sight.
- You will be given eye drops (these sting a bit for a few seconds) which make the pupils of your eyes bigger to allow the retina at the back of the eye to be photographed. After 15 minutes your vision will become blurred and it will be difficult to focus on objects near you. THIS IS NORMAL so don't worry. Your vision will go back to normal again (effects last from 2–6 hours, depending on the drops used). THIS MEANS YOU CAN'T DRIVE HOME AFTERWARDS.
- You will be seated in front of a machine that takes a photograph of the retina of each eye. The camera DOES NOT touch your eyes. You will see a flash of light for each photograph taken. The light is bright but this is a painless procedure and you shouldn't feel uncomfortable.

You should take your glasses with you and take a pair of sunglasses for afterwards as you will find your eyes are sensitive to light because your pupils have been enlarged. If, like me, you wear contact lenses, you will need to remove them so the camera can photograph your retinas (so take our lens pot with you). You can put your lenses back in afterwards, but you may want to give your eyes a rest and wear glasses instead (if you have them).

FACT: You should not drive to and from your eye screening appointment.

Very rarely the eye drops can cause a rapid increase in pressure in the eyes. THIS ONLY HAPPENS in people who are already at risk of developing this problem. If this happens it will be treated quickly in the eye unit. The symptoms of high pressure in the eyes are:

- Pain or severe discomfort in your eyes.
- Redness of the white of your eyes.
- Blurred sight, sometimes with rainbow halos around lights.

FACT: If you experience any of these symptoms after screening you should return to the eye unit or go to the hospital Accident and Emergency department.

After your eye screening your retinal photographs may have to be seen by an eye specialist or more than one health professional, so you won't get the results straight away. You will be told how long it will be before you get your written results and if you are not told this information, make sure you ask. The results will also be sent to your GP and to the National Screening Programme. No one else will see your results unless you give them permission. You may want to take a copy of your screening results to give to your diabetes team. You may be called back to the screening centre if:

- They find sight-threatening retinopathy needing follow-up treatment from the hospital eye clinic.
- The photographs are unclear and don't give an accurate result.
- The level of retinopathy you have needs to be monitored more often than once a year.
- Other eye conditions are found during the screening process that need more investigation.

If you are worried about or have problems with your eyes in between eye screening appointments, such as sudden loss or worsening of vision; blurring of vision that doesn't go away and this is not because of sudden sustained improvement in BG levels (this can cause temporary worsening of sight); distorted vision; a sudden increase in 'floaters' in your vision; or part of your vision appears to be missing or obscured – DON'T WAIT FOR YOUR NEXT SCREENING APPOINTMENT – SEEK PROFESSIONAL ADVICE.

The screening unit will keep your photographs for at least eight years so they can compare future ones and detect changes over time. A small number of retinal photographs undergo quality control tests to make sure they have been properly assessed. You can reduce your risk of developing sight-threatening eye changes by:

- Keeping your BG levels within normal range (aim for between 5–7 mmol/L).
- Making sure your blood pressure is monitored regularly.

- Attending regular eye screening appointments.

- Attending regular diabetes checks.

- Having your blood fats (lipids and cholesterol) checked regularly.

- Don't smoke.

NERVE DISEASE

Unfortunately, high BG levels often take their toll on the nervous system in the form of neuropathy (nerve damage) and 60% of people diagnosed with diabetes will experience this. This complication is usually seen in people who have had diabetes for many years, those over 40, and in people who smoke. There are two kinds: *peripheral neuropathy*, affecting the feet and hands; and *autonomic neuropathy*, where there is damage to the nerves that control actions we don't have to think about, like breathing, heartbeat, digestive function, and the bladder muscles.

Case Study

Christina Santos had both peripheral and autonomic neuropathies because her Type 2 diabetes had been poorly controlled for over twenty years. She described the problems in her lower legs and feet as flashing pains, heavy legs, numbness, extreme sensitivity to touch, and muscle tenderness. She also had no knee or ankle reflexes. She had developed several foot ulcers over the years and amputation had been threatened because of both her nerve damage and poor blood supply. Christina was told that the damage was irreversible, so she continued to eat whatever she liked and did not take her diabetes medication regularly. She also had problems with autonomic neuropathy because of long-term high BG levels. She developed gastroparesis (delayed stomach emptying) which meant that the rate at which she digested food was very slow because her stomach did not empty at the normal rate. This caused many more problems with high blood glucose levels because the medication she was taking was not working at the same time as when her meals were digested. Christina also suffered other side-effects of gastro-intestinal nerve damage such as abdominal bloating, wind, pain, and severe diarrhoea.

FACT: Approximately one in six people with diabetes develop a foot ulcer at some time in their life.

You may have had tests done when you visit your diabetes clinic to see if there are any signs of nerve damage in your feet. These include tests to see if you can feel vibrations, temperature changes and light touch testing to see if you can sense something touching your skin. If your consultant finds that you do not feel certain sensations in response to these tests, a diagnosis of peripheral neuropathy will be made. This may either be SENSORY nerve damage; MOTOR nerve damage (these carry impulses to muscles to make them move); or AUTONOMIC nerve damage. Some people with neuropathy may not have all of the usual symptoms, or symptoms such as abdominal bloating and diahorrea can be mistaken for irritable bowel syndrome instead of autonomic neuropathy as it is very difficult to diagnose. Below you can find a list of disorders associated with neuropathy:

Sensation problems
These are very common in people with diabetes and either affect many nerves in the body or only a few. DISTAL POLYNEUROPATHY affects many of the nerves in the feet and hands and is caused by high BG levels over time. The symptoms of polyneuropathy are:

- Reduced ability to feel light touch and lack of awareness of the position of the foot.
- Reduced pain and temperature sensations.
- Tingling and burning sensations. Weakness.
- Sensations like walking on pebbles.
- Increased sensitivity to touch.
- Loss of balance and/or co-ordination.
- These symptoms are often worse during the night.

FACT: The good news is there are two medications designed to help with neuropathy (nerve damage) symptoms. *Gabapentin* (Neurontin) reduces neuropathy pain, allowing better sleep; and *Memantine*, which doesn't have any known side-effects.

Case Study

David Lynn was 49 with Type 1 diabetes for 30 years. Although he had improved his BG control over the past 10 years, earlier nerve damage had led to neuropathy in his legs, feet and hands. These areas of his body were numb and cold, although he had a good blood supply in both feet. David tended to walk around the house barefoot and one day he trod on one of his son's Lego bricks. He felt some discomfort but thought no more of it. A week later David's wife, Lynn, noticed he was limping slightly. She examined his foot and found he had split the skin on the sole which had become infected. Lynn cleaned the wound and put a dressing on it. David went to his GP and, to his surprise, was told he would have to go into hospital. Because people with diabetes have slow wound healing, David remained in hospital for two weeks as the wound was intensively treated with antibiotic powder. David was not allowed to walk on the foot for a month and he was discharged from hospital on crutches. David now always makes sure he wears slippers indoors and checks his feet every day.

There are also other serious problems that can develop in the feet associated with long-term high BG levels. FOOT ULCERS are a very serious complication that can happen because of loss of feeling in the feet. Normal areas of pressure on the feet cannot be detected as pain and an area of hard skin develops. Over time this continued pressure on this hardened skin causes it to break down and soften until it becomes mushy and comes away, leaving a deep hole, or ulcer in the foot that becomes infected. If professional help is not sought for a diabetic foot ulcer, the hole becomes larger and the blood supply dies off. At this stage the only thing that can be done is to amputate (possibly the whole of the lower leg) to save the person's life.

Another serious foot problem can happen if a person with diabetes injures their foot but doesn't feel it. The small foot bones can be moved out of position and multiple pain-free fractures occur. The foot and ankle swell up and become red and the foot eventually becomes useless. This condition is called *neuroarthropathy* (also known as CHARCOT JOINTS).

Case Study

Eva Gomez was 29 and had experienced really difficult to control Type 1 diabetes since she was 10 years old. One morning Eva woke up and the whole of her left foot was swollen to three times the size of her right. The foot didn't hurt, and Eva couldn't afford to miss work, so she put on a pair of roomy boots and hobbled to her job as an Administrator. The next day Eva's foot was no better. She did not have a good relationship with her diabetes consultant because he would warn her about her poor BG control, although he didn't have any solutions to offer her. Eva continued to walk around and, after 18 months, her foot finally went back to normal size. Eva was horrified to find that her left foot was now much wider across the bridge than her right. Her big toe had dislocated downwards and her third and fourth toes were now bent and misshapen. She also had a large area of hard skin on her sole beneath the third and fourth toe. Eva now wishes she had gone to see her doctor when she first found her foot was swollen. As she walks, although there is no pain, her foot now makes a crunching sound as the bones grind and Eva can now only wear flat, orthopaedic shoes.

FACT: Good, regular foot care can reduce amputation rates by 45–85%.

Movement problems

Diabetes also affects the nerves and muscles that allow us to move around easily because of changes to their blood supply. Any of our nerves may be affected and, unfortunately the only way to prevent this complication is with good BG control. For those people who have extreme difficulty in achieving good BG results (like me) the best control possible with insulin pump therapy is sometimes not enough to overcome many years of poor BG control meaning associated nerve damage is inevitable.

Autonomic nerve problems

As I mentioned earlier, autonomic nerve damage affects nerve and muscle functions that go on in the body all the time. Problems caused by poor BG control over time can show themselves in a number of ways:

The HEART may not pump more blood to the muscles when it is needed, such as when standing up from a sitting position, causing light headedness. The heart rate may also be very fast and/or the heart rhythm may become disrupted, increasing the chance of sudden death. When there is autonomic nerve damage the resting heart rate is high, blood pressure drops very low when standing, and the general heart rate when breathing in and out is low. The heart may also become larger (*cardiomyopathy*) and is unable to pump enough blood, leading to a faster heart rate and problems if there is already a high blood pressure.

The LARGE INTESTINE can be affected dramatically by autonomic neuropathy, where there is ongoing and frequent diarrhoea, and loss of bowel control. This can be treated with medication to stop the need for such frequent visits to the toilet, but there may also be alternate diarrhoea and constipation. If the stomach nerves are damaged the time taken to digest food slows down, causing problems with matching BG-lowering doses with BG ups and downs. Insulin pump therapy helps match rates of digestion to insulin needs in Type 1 diabetes and a medication called *metocloprimide* helps the stomach to empty more quickly.

The GALL BLADDER can develop gallstones due to nerve damage so that it doesn't empty properly after eating, especially if the meal has a high fat content. Bile (produced by the body to break down fat) builds up and hardens in the gall bladder to form gall stones.

If the BLADDER nerves become damaged there is loss of awareness of when the bladder is full. This leads to urine tract infections, urine does not flow normally but dribbles out, and a person with this problem may have to strain to push urine out of the bladder. Medication can increase the force of the bladder muscles when they contract to release urine and attempting to urinate every four hours can avoid infections.

As previously mentioned, problems with SEXUAL FUNCTION are experienced by 50% of men with diabetes (*erectile dysfunction*) and one-third of females (vaginal dryness).

The nerves of the PUPILS OF THE EYES may be affected by autonomic neuropathy, meaning thy cannot adjust to let in more or less light when needed.

Although you might not realise it, EXCESSIVE SWEATING may be down to your diabetes. People with diabetes may find that the skin on their feet is dry because the feet don't sweat, but the face and upper body sweat profusely to compensate. People have also reported that eating foods like cheese cause them to sweat very heavily.

As well as nerve damage to the heart in diabetes, high BG levels have the potential to cause CORONARY HEART DISEASE where the blood supply becomes gradually less and less. This is due to narrowing of the coronary arteries supplying the heart and this is something that happens over time in people with Type 1 diabetes. Heart disease happens much more quickly in people with Type 2 diabetes because BG levels can be abnormally high for as long as 12 years (according to Diabetes UK) before diabetes is finally diagnosed. Meanwhile, high glucose levels cause the arteries to fur up.

Other factors that increase the risk of heart disease in Type 2 diabetes or pre-diabetes (the same thing as insulin resistance – defined as blood glucose concentrations higher than normal, but lower than established limits for diabetes itself) are having high blood pressure; high blood fats (such as cholesterol); insulin resistance; obesity, especially fat around the waist; and smoking.

VASCULAR DISEASE occurs when the blood vessels in the hands and feet become blocked – this happens at an earlier age in people with diabetes than in the general population who do not have diabetes. Because of vascular disease, after a decade one-third of people with diabetes will have lost the arterial pulses in their feet. This complication of diabetes affects multiple arteries in the body and this may happen because of things you can't do anything about, such as for genetic reasons, becoming older, and having diabetes. BUT there are things you can do to slow down this damage to the main blood vessels: reducing your HbA1c level (the amount of glucose sticking to red blood cells over their lifetime); stopping smoking; reducing your blood cholesterol level; managing high blood pressure levels; and controlling your body weight.

As I've mentioned, ALL arteries and blood vessels are damaged by high BG levels, including those of the BRAIN. If the arteries supplying the brain with oxygen become blocked there are serious consequences. A partial restriction in blood supply (*transient ischaemia*) results in a mini-stroke with slurring of speech, muscle weakness down one side of the body, and numbness. This frightening situation may last for a few minutes, hours or days depending on how much of the artery is blocked. If the artery closes completely due to the formation of a large blood clot, a full stroke occurs. The good news is, the quicker a stroke sufferer gets professional help, the sooner treatment to dissolve the blood clot can be given. This is the reason that people with diabetes are prescribed small daily doses of aspirin to thin the blood and prevent clots.

OTHER CONSEQUENCES OF SURVIVING WITH DIABETES are joint and muscle pain. This is because diabetes affects all body systems, including muscle and bone. Some joint conditions are difficult to confirm as diabetes-related as they're similar to problems experienced by the general population:

Case Study

Dev Mobarak was in his mid-forties with Type 2 diabetes when he began experiencing severe shoulder pain, limited movement and stiffness. His GP diagnosed a frozen shoulder and sent Dev for intense physiotherapy to loosen the joint and reduce the pain. Dev found these physio sessions incredibly painful and sought a second opinion with a private doctor specialising in joint conditions. Dev was diagnosed with *shoulder adhesive capsulitis* and he was told this was a severe complication caused by very high BG levels. It limited the movement in his arm because the surface of the shoulder joint had thickened and connective tissue had stuck to the head of the humerus bone. The physiotherapy prescribed due to misdiagnosis had pulled these abnormal connections in Dev's shoulder, causing more pain. Dev improved his BG control and found the pain was reduced, although the adhesions were permanent, so he was left with limited movement.

THE HANDS of people with diabetes may become stiff, painful and swollen, reducing movement as the small bones are affected. This is seen in as many as 50% of people with Type 1 or Type 2 diabetes. CARPAL TUNNEL SYNDROME (where the tendons in the hands and wrists shorten so the finger rest in a claw-like position), is common in association with diabetes, as is DUPUYTREN'S DISEASE (where the tendons of the wrists shorten and the palms become thickened so they cannot be placed together in a prayer-like position.

THE VERTEBRA (spinal joints) may join together in a condition known as *hyperstosis*, limiting movement in obese people with Type 2 diabetes. Gout and *osteoarthritis* is common in the bones of the feet, especially in association with obesity where the feet have to support a greater weight. A condition where there's lack of bone mass (*osteopenia*) is also seen in people with Type 1 diabetes.

FACT: Diabetes is associated with many joint and connective tissue disorders.

Some skin conditions only appear in people with diabetes and can actually be a warning sign that complications will develop. This is the case because of changes to the small blood vessels and an increase in collagen (the protein found in cartilage and bone) is commonly seen in all complications. As we have already seen, DRY SKIN is a problem associated with peripheral neuropathy in the feet due to a lack of sweating, whilst thickened skin in diabetes is due to an increase in collagen. VITILIGO (loss of skin pigmentation) happens in people with Type1 diabetes as part of the auto-immune (self-attack) process.

A skin condition seen in Indian, Hispanic and black populations, ACANTHOSIS NIGRICANS, causes velvety areas of dark pigmentation to form on the back of the neck and armpits. This condition can be improved with weight loss and the application of vitamin A and vitamin D creams. A diabetes-related skin condition, NECROBIOSIS LIPOIDICA, is seen more frequently in women, where reddish-brown patches of skin form mostly on the shins and ankles, although it can also occur on the upper limbs, upper body and face. Another skin problem seen more often in people with diabetes, is XANTHELASMA where small yellow fat deposits develop on the eyelids and other areas of skin. This can be an indicator that blood fats are high, so if these develop, go to your GP for blood tests to check fat levels. This condition can also be associated with inflammation of the pancreas and this can lead to diabetes (if you don't already have it) because swelling changes the organ's ability to work properly. As with all complications of diabetes, treatment for xanthelasma involves tightening BG control.

FACT: Diabetes does not just affect your body physically – it can also affect your mental health.

As we saw earlier, BG levels are hugely affected by our emotions. Not surprisingly, diabetes has a great impact on mental wellbeing because of the continual self-management demands as we try to delay or stabilise the chronic complications listed previously. DEPRESSION is three-times more likely to develop in people with diabetes than in people without diabetes, although its cause is unknown. What is known is that a number of factors contribute towards the development of depression, although it can often remain unrecognised and undiagnosed. The major difficulty with depression is that it leads to poor motivation for diabetes self-care, so necessary activities like insulin injection or glucose medication-taking, regular blood testing and exercise can be ignored, especially if depression is severe.

Depression can also lead to higher BG levels due to hormonal and chemical changes in the body, and it can reoccur throughout a person's lifetime. Women tend to develop depression more often than men, and there are similar rates in people with Type 1 and Type 2 diabetes. There are a number of symptoms – some of which you may not think of as depression: not being able to sleep; feeling muddled because you can't think clearly; having little or no energy; getting easily upset and feeling like you aren't a worthwhile person; you may not feel like eating or you may over-eat to cheer yourself up; you don't feel like doing the normal activities you usually enjoy; you lose your sense of humour; and you feel like you can't go on. Depression can be treated with anti-depressant medication, or with psychotherapy (such as 'talking therapies'). Both work just as well, with 50–60% of people seeing an improvement in their symptoms after three months of treatment.

Case Study

Judith Dixon was 33 when she had her first episode of severe depression. Her GP did not say that it would affect her diabetes in any way, but Judith found she could not meet the demands of trying to keep her BG under control. She had no interest in her usual social activities, so she gave up her keep fit classes and cycling with her friends at weekends. She also lost interest in caring for herself, and stopped caring about her hygiene or changing her clothes. She became so withdrawn she rarely left the house. Judith couldn't explain why she felt the way she did but after two months, Judith's sister Sandra decided to make another appointment with the GP and this time, Sandra went along to explain how Judith's depression was actually affecting her life. The GP prescribed some anti-depressants, but these had unpleasant side effects so Sandra took Judith to see her GP for a third time. She was prescribed a course of Cognitive Behavioural Therapy to help her recognise how her thoughts affected her feelings and behaviour. After 16 sessions of this treatment, Judith's severe depression finally lifted.

Prevention of complications

As I've mentioned throughout the section on complications, the best way to stop them from developing, or stop them from getting worse if you already have, for example, diabetic eye disease or nerve problems, is to aim to keep your BG tests between 5–7 mmol/L, this meaning your HbA1c is as near the normal 6% (42 mmol/L) as possible. This is easier said than done and can be practically impossible if you have dramatic swings in your BG. Regular BG tests give you the information to see when you might need more or less insulin, or when your glucose medication is reducing your BG too much or not enough. It's important to work closely with your GP and diabetes consultant and nurse to get the best possible control of your BG. Preventing the onset of complications is the best possible motivation for good BG management.

Case Study

Ellie Schaffer developed Type 1 diabetes when she was eight and took her condition very seriously. When Ellie was 24, her mother, Jan (also with Type 1), died from diabetes-related heart disease. Her mother had always been Ellie's motivation for looking after herself because, over the years, she also saw her mother go blind and have three toes amputated from her left foot because she didn't want to look after her diabetes.

Case Study

Lucy King had been taking insulin for a couple of years to treat her Type 2 diabetes. She never felt completely in control of her BG levels until she decided to keep a diary of her results. This helped her see patterns forming when she was higher or lower than she wanted. After a couple of weeks Lucy realised she needed more insulin in the mornings and that she tended to dip down with much lower BG levels in the afternoon. She changed her insulin dosages accordingly and found her next HbA1c was 6.5% (48 mmol/L).

FACT: Having diabetes means lower limb amputation is 15 to 70 times more likely.

This is a very scary statistic BUT your diabetes consultant and your GP will regularly ask to see your feet to check for any diabetic changes; in the same way your urine will be checked for protein and your eyes will be tested to ensure there are no problems developing. As masters of our own diabetes, we are in the best position to know when something isn't quite right. It is also a very good idea if you check your own feet every day for cuts, blisters or sore patches, and report any problems and changes you notice in any part of your body as soon as possible to your GP. Foot care for people with diabetes is a priority and there are many chiropody and podiatry services (specialising in foot care) available that you can visit or that will even come to you if you have mobility problems.

FACT: Foot problems in people with diabetes are the most preventable complication because changes like numbness or areas of hard skin can be detected quickly by YOU and can be speedily treated by your health care team.

EXERCISING WITH FOOT PROBLEMS

You may not think you have any problems with your feet, especially if you have no symptoms or pain, tingling, burning or numbness, or any areas of pressure and callouses that could become foot ulcers. Even if this is the case IT'S IMPORTANT as I've already mentioned, to check your feet CAREFULLY every day for any changes. If you do have any diabetic changes, this is not an excuse to avoid exercising – you just have to make sure you exercise in a way that is appropriate and that won't make your foot problems worse. REMEMBER if you have any loss of sensation (numbness) in your feet you may not feel an injury:

- Make sure you change your footwear every five hours and don't wear tight trainers or shoes to exercise in as they will restrict the blood flow. A pair of cushioned trainers or a roomy pair (but not loose so they rub up and down) with gel insoles inserted makes a good choice of footwear.
- Make sure you don't wear socks with seams or holes that can rub part of your foot and cause a blister or a wound.
- If you do find an injury, blister, bruise or any other type of change when you remove your trainers, see a health professional as soon as possible to have it treated.

WHAT ELSE CAN I DO TO PROTECT MY FEET?
- Make sure your shoes, or even the seams on your socks, aren't rubbing and that your shoes aren't tight.
- Don't walk without something on your feet.
- Shock absorbing gel insoles can make a big difference by relieving pressure and foot pain.
- Make sure you don't have anything in your shoes, such as gravel from outside, BEFORE you put them on.
- Don't use hard skin removal 'sanding' machines with spinning pumice stone, revolving toenail buffer/sanding devices; heated foot pads or vibrating foot massage machines.
- If you have problems finding shoes that fit, ask you GP, diabetes team or podiatrist for a referral to an ORTOTIST at the hospital. This is a specially-trained person who can make you made-to-measure shoes that will fit you perfectly so they won't rub and cause problems.

- DIABETES AND SMOKING DON'T MIX – it clogs up blood vessels and reduces blood flow, increasing the risk of amputation.
- Wash and moisturise your feet daily. DO NOT use hot water and dry thoroughly before adding the cream – THIS IS A MUST if the skin on your feet is very dry.
- If you do notice areas of pressure on your feet, stop wearing shoes that cause pressure.
- If you develop an area of skin on your foot that becomes infected (red around the edges, hot to the touch and 'squishy' or if pus has formed), inform your GP as soon as possible, raise the foot and rest it – don't be tempted to walk on it!

Case Study

I once knelt down to do some painting of a skirting board and felt one of my toes go crack with the pressure of taking my weight in this position. I didn't feel any pain but found, after having it investigated, that I had broken my toe. So BE CAREFUL of putting any pressure on your toe joints by crouching down or stretching upwards on tip-toe.

The effects of certain medications and other health conditions on your BG

As I've mentioned before, people with diabetes often need more of certain vitamins as deficiencies can affect BG and hormone levels. The proper production of adrenal hormones, insulin (in Type 2 diabetes) and a substance known as glucose tolerance factor by the liver rely on good levels of vitamins C, B3, B5, B6, zinc and chromium. Because insulin is a hormone, it is affected by other levels of hormones, certain medications and other medical problems that you may also have.

MEDICATIONS & NUTRITIONAL SUPPLEMENTS THAT INCREASE BG

Both prescribed medications and over-the-counter products can have a marked effect on your BG levels. *Statins* (prescribed to reduce cholesterol levels) have been in the news lately because people who take these tablets have a higher risk of developing Type 2 diabetes as they raise BG levels, as well as increasing BG for those who already have Type 2. If you do take statins, it's advisable to carry on doing so because the risk of heart disease and stroke from having high cholesterol levels without statins is greater than an increase in BG when you take them. *Vitamin B3* (also known as nicotinic acid) reduces insulin production, affecting people with Type 2 diabetes by raising BG levels. This may be taken in a vitamin supplement or be prescribed by your GP to treat a high cholesterol level.

Thiazide tablets (or diuretics – 'water tablets') also have a tendency to increase BG levels because they reduce potassium levels in the body meaning insulin is less able to work to reduce BG levels. This is also the case for some tablets taken for high blood pressure (*Attenolol, Bisopropol, Minoxidil, Nifedipine,* and *Amlodipine*) that alter the way glucose is processed by the body.

Some *Corticosteroid* tablets prescribed for inflammatory conditions, and even some steroid creams used to treat and manage skin conditions like eczema, can increase BG levels. Some tablets taken to prevent organ rejection following transplant (such as *Prednisone*) increase BG levels because they destroy the insulin-producing cells of the pancreas, meaning more insulin is needed in people with Type 2 diabetes. Drug treatments for psychosis (severe mental disorder where thoughts and emotions are impaired) such as *Chlorpromazine*, *Promazine*, *Fluphennazine* and *Tripfluoperazine* also reduce insulin production meaning that BG levels are increased.

MEDICATIONS & NUTRITIONAL SUPPLEMENTS THAT CAN DECREASE BG

Certain forms of antibiotics and some water tablets (diuretics) have the same effect. Some corticosteroids can reduce BG levels (always check the leaflet that comes with your prescription or over-the-counter medications). This is also the case for recreational drugs like heroin, and sleeping pills like barbiturates. *Alpha blockers* (such as *Doxazpsin* derivatives) that are used to treat high blood pressure also have the effect of lowering BG, as do *fibric acid* derivatives (used to treat fat disorders).

It is known that people who take fish oil supplements and aspirin at the same time can suffer from hypoglycaemia. Aspirin stops the absorption of glucose in the small intestine and Omega 3 fish oils have the same effect meaning that frequent low BG levels can result. Aspirin also increases the effects of some BG-lowering medications taken to treat Type 2 diabetes. Oil of Evening Primrose capsules interfere with the way BG-lowering medication works in people taking tablets and insulin to manage their diabetes, with the effect that it lowers BG levels.

FACT: A nutritional supplement that can IMPROVE eye health by reducing cell damage at the back of the eye is a combination of lutein and zeaxanthin. I take 20 milligrams once

**a day and my vision is sharper, eye 'floaters' (black specks)
have decreased or disappeared, and I have better night vision.**

MEDICAL CONDITIONS THAT ARE ASSOCIATED WITH HIGH
BG LEVELS

Other than diabetes itself, there are several chronic long-term
medical conditions that have an effect on BG levels, making them
higher. *Coeliac disease* is a chronic auto-immune condition
triggered by an intolerance to gluten (a protein found in cereal
grains such as wheat that is added to bread to make it rise) causing
inflammation of the small bowel in the intestines. This condition is
treated with a gluten-free diet, but gluten-free foods contain more
carbohydrate than foods like bread made with gluten added. This
additional carbohydrate in the gluten-free version increases BG
levels more than the gluten-added version, meaning more insulin is
needed.

There are several auto-immune conditions affecting the
thyroid gland: *hypothyroidism* (an under-active thyroid gland);
Graves' disease (an enlarged and over-active thyroid gland); and
Hashimoto's thyroiditis (a condition causing the thyroid to produce
less thyroid hormone). Too much thyroid hormone causes insulin to
work for a shorter time and to be less effective at reducing BG.
Increased levels of thyroid hormone causes the body to produce
more glucose. (The body's use of carbohydrate is also affected if
there is not enough thyroid hormone so the liver produces LESS
glucose, reducing BG levels and increasing the risk of hypos.)
Although having an under-active thyroid usually results in low BG
levels, some people (myself included) find that they have
unexplained higher BG levels as a result:

Case Study

Wendy Payne had Type 1 diabetes for 25 years when she was told she also had an under-active thyroid gland after routine blood tests. Wendy had been tired and had no energy for a long time and her brain seemed very slow. Her GP started her on a low dose of thyroxin but she didn't feel any different. Wendy had blood tests every three months and was told each time that the condition was getting worse. Her own BG tests were up and down without explanation and her diabetes consultant felt Wendy wasn't looking after herself properly. He warned her that her mild sight problems would get more serious if she didn't do more to help herself. Wendy felt it wasn't her fault and read as much as she could about thyroid problems. Wendy told her consultant that an under-active thyroid gland could cause high BG levels, but he disagreed with her that this was the problem. Eventually Wendy's BG levels stabilised when she was put on a higher dose of thyroid hormone, proving Wendy was right.

Psoriasis is an auto-immune condition that affects the skin and joints. It is now recognised that psoriasis is associated with an increase in the production of insulin, increasing BG levels and leading to the later development of Type 2 diabetes. Obesity (defined as a body mass index of 30 and above) increases the risk of developing moderate to severe psoriasis, and psoriasis has also been linked to the factors common in the development of Type 2 diabetes such the body not being able to manage glucose levels well. This means that psoriasis is more likely to develop when there is insulin resistance.

MEDICAL CONDITIONS THAT ARE ASSOCIATED WITH LOW BG LEVELS

As well as under-active thyroid conditions that may result in lower BG levels, other auto-immune conditions can reduce BG levels. *Addison's disease* affects the adrenal glands (on top of the kidneys) and this condition can cause frequent and severe hypoglycaemia (low BG levels) because it affects hormones that maintain the amount of glucose in the blood. A rare non-cancerous tumour of the pancreas, called an *insulinoma*, secretes insulin and causes unexplained hypoglycaemia. Severe infections, such as *pneumonia*, have the effect of reducing BG levels by making the body use up more glucose in response to fighting the infection. Diseases like *malaria* can stimulate the body to produce more insulin.

Auto-immune syndrome causes there to be a large amount of insulin in the bloodstream despite BG already being low. Mostly, this insulin is inactive, but this situation can reverse. *Hereditary fructose disorder* causes low BG levels in children because their bodies can't use the sugars found in fruit. *Glycogen storage disease* is a condition where there is slow release of glucose by the liver and resulting hypoglycaemia. People with this problem are advised to eat slow-release carbohydrates like oats and bread so that their BG levels don't rise too quickly after a meal. People with liver, kidney or glandular diseases might fund they have low BG levels because use of glucose by the body is increased by these conditions. Hypoglycaemia may also happen if a person suffers a long and severe lack of oxygen.

DIET & EXERCISE

'It's not easy and it takes a lot of self-control, but it's definitely worth it'

There are educational courses available for people with Type 1 or Type 2 diabetes to help them manage their condition in the best possible way. Whatever type of diabetes you have, your GP, Practice Nurse or Diabetes Nurse will recommend the course that is appropriate to you and they will book you a place to attend at a venue that's local to you.

FACT: Most people with diabetes only get 3 hours a year with their GP, diabetes consultant and diabetes nurse – the rest of the time it's down to us to self-manage diabetes.

Making friends with DAFNE if you have Type 1 diabetes

For people with Type 1 diabetes who take insulin, the opportunity is there to live a virtually normal life eating what you like, when you like. This, of course, depends on knowing how much carbohydrate is contained in the food you want to eat, how much insulin is required for that carbohydrate, and how and when it will work to lower your BG so your levels stay within normal limits. The rate at which you digest food is also a factor. Autonomic nerve damage can slow down the rate of digestion so it takes many hours making it difficult to match insulin needs, leading to hypos – when there is not enough food available for insulin to work on; then high BG levels once the insulin has worked but food is now available, raising BG levels.

DAFNE – What does this mean?

DAFNE stands for Dosage Adjustment For Normal Eating. DAFNE is an educational course for people with type 1 diabetes to give them the skills they need to administer the right amount of insulin for the amount of carbohydrate they choose to eat. Carbohydrate counting used to be a method emphasised by health professionals to control what you ate (this is the method I was taught in the 1970s). This way of thinking then fell out of favour but it's now back again with the new approach that you count carbohydrates and have appropriate insulin to allow freedom in your lifestyle and food choices.

HOW LONG does the DAFNE course last?

DAFNE is a course lasting for 5 days. There is a one-day follow up after 8 weeks to allow you to discuss your experiences and any problems you may have experienced.

HOW MANY PEOPLE WILL BE ON THE COURSE WITH ME?

The course is designed to involve a small group of 6 people with Type 1 diabetes. You can participate in discussions and share your experiences with the group and/or speak to the DAFNE trainer in private.

IS IT WORTH ME GOING AS I CAN ALREADY ALTER MY INSULIN?

Although you may already be altering your insulin and having more if you eat a big meal, the DAFNE course also offers vital information, education and support that really can help you to manage your BG levels to improve your diabetes control.

CAN I GO ON A DAFNE COURSE IF I HAVE TYPE 2 DIABETES?

Even if you use insulin to treat your Type 2 diabetes, the DAFNE course is designed for people with Type 1, which is a different form of diabetes and requires different management techniques to Type 2 diabetes. For these reasons, the DAFNE course is not offered to people with Type 2 diabetes.

Because people with Type 1 diabetes don't tend to be overweight, the aim of DAFNE is to be able to eat normally by calculating carbohydrate and necessary insulin dosages to keep BG levels normal. People with Type 2 diabetes taking insulin do so because their BG levels are not controlled as well by glucose-reducing medication. The aim for people with Type 2 diabetes is to control their BG levels by losing weight and cutting down on carbohydrates such as cakes, sweets, chocolate, pies, biscuits, crisps and chips.

WILL GOING ON THIS COURSE MAKE A BIG CHANGE IN MY LIFE?

One of the aims of the course is to help people accommodate diabetes into their lifestyle more easily so that THEY CONTROL THEIR DIABETES, rather than IT CONTROLLING THEM. This means that making your insulin dosages appropriate for what you eat will be made as simple as possible so you don't have to make huge changes to the way you do things at the moment.

WHAT WILL I LEARN ON THE COURSE?

The course covers all aspects of food and taking insulin:

- How to count carbohydrate portions.

- How to set a background insulin dose (insulin that works all the time to keep your BG within normal range).
- How to take bolus insulin dosages (the insulin you give for meals, or when you have to bring down a high BG).
- How to correct BG levels when they are too high or too low.
- Managing BG levels and exercise.

Case Study

Justin Moore was 26 and had been struggling with his Type 1 diabetes for almost 10 years. He checked his BG up to 10 times a day and gave himself insulin if he was high, but he didn't know how much insulin he should be taking, and he usually ended up hypo a few hours later. He also always had a hypo if he tried to take any exercise. Eventually Justin's diabetes consultant referred him for the DAFNE course when he realised that Justin's lifestyle was ruled by his diabetes. After attending the course, he felt he had a good understanding of how his diabetes affected him, what his BG results actually meant and how to act on them, and how his insulin was working. Justin was given step-by-step practical solutions to BG problems and five months later his BG control is excellent – he rarely has a hypo and he knows exactly what he's doing with carbs and insulin rather than guessing.

FACT: Not every diabetes centre can offer the DAFNE course because this needs specially-trained educators. If it's not available in your area, you can sign up to do the DAFNE course online at http://www.dafne.uk.com

IF YOU HAVE TYPE 2

As we saw earlier, there are lifestyle changes we can all make to help reduce BG levels and the risk of developing serious complications. These include increasing the amount of physical activity you do each day; choosing healthy foods over high fat, high calorie ones; understanding your prescribed medications – what they're for, when to take them and how much; and working with the health professionals who look after you. Each of these challenges can be difficult but you don't have to face them on your own, for example, if you exercise with friends or eat with family.

As with any major changes you need to make in your life, it's best if you start gradually. If you try to do it all at once, you will find it overwhelming and you'll be more likely to give up. START BY DOING LITTLE THINGS THAT WILL MAKE A BIG DIFFERENCE like swapping sugary drinks for diet or sugar-free ones; reducing or stopping adding sugar to the hot drinks and meals you make at home; and reducing the amount of sweet snacks like biscuits, cake and chocolate that you eat each day. Like any habit, this new way of managing your diet will take time to become something you do without even thinking about it.

FACT: It takes 21 days (3 weeks) to break a bad habit such as eating a daily bar of chocolate. Forming a new habit like eating a piece of fruit every day takes 66 days (3 months) to establish.

In the same way as making different food choices, you could make changes to the amount of physical activity you do if you are able to by making the choice to walk rather than drive if it's for a short distance; by walking for longer (involve your dog in your new exercise routine if you have one!); and climbing stairs rather than using an escalator or lift if possible. These are just general suggestions and you must decide what is an achievable goal for you. Remember, having Type 2 diabetes is a health condition that you CAN do something about if you make changes to your lifestyle.

Getting to know DESMOND if you have Type 2 diabetes

DESMOND – What does this mean?

DESMOND stands for Diabetes Education and Self-Management for Ongoing and Newly Diagnosed. This is a course recommended by your GP or Practice Nurse that's run by experts in Type 2 diabetes. It's run by nurses, dieticians and diabetes educators and it's designed to help you understand and get to grips with your diagnosis and gives you useful information about how to manage your diabetes. At the DESMOND course you will meet other people who have also just recently been diagnosed with Type 2 diabetes and the course leaders will encourage you to talk about any worries you have about looking after yourself.

Case Study

Doreen Brown was in her early seventies when her GP told her that she had Type 2 diabetes. Doreen was very shocked as she had not felt unwell. It also seemed silly to her to start worrying about changing what she ate and doing more exercise. Doreen was invited to attend the DESMOND course and she went along, expecting it to be of little interest to her. Doreen was surprised to find a small, friendly group of people attending the course who had the same feelings and worries and they shared ideas and offered support. She found out how to make sensible food choices and why it was important to make an effort to improve her health. She began to change the portion sizes of her meals, eating half as any potatoes every day and cutting out biscuits. She still made her own cakes but Doreen cut the sugar in the recipe by two-thirds. When Doreen had another diabetes check three months later at her GP surgery she was told that her condition was so much improved her BG was normal.

It's a good idea to write down anything you want to ask. Because you are going into a new situation and you have many things on your mind, you may forget what you wanted to say as your brain can be relied upon to fail to remind you. With questions written down before you go to the DESMOND course, you will feel calm and ready to start learning. The course will focus mainly on food groups and how these affect your BG. Changes in diet are always of more benefit when you also make changes to improve your physical activity levels.

ASSESSING YOUR PHYSICAL ACTIVITY

As we've already seen, keeping active helps manage BG levels in a big way. You might think you are fairly active already because, for example, you walk your dog every day, or you go up and down the stairs at home several times a day. Being physically active is unique to each individual – if you have always done a physical job like building work then this is obviously different to an older retired person who has arthritis and cannot move around much. The key is, increasing the amount of activity YOU do each day if you can. This doesn't mean that you have to join a gym or start jogging around the park every morning. It can be bending and flexing your legs at the knees or lifting your arms up and down while you are sitting watching television.

FACT: Every movement BURNS GLUCOSE and strengthening your muscles when you have diabetes is very important to maintain movement and good mobility.

As with how many portions of fruit and vegetables we should eat a day there are recommendations about physical activity. Obviously not everyone can manage what's recommended because they have physical disabilities where what should be done isn't possible. We are told to do 30 minutes of MODERATELY INTENSIVE activity (meaning we get warmer and our breathing is increased as heart rate is faster) at least 5 times a week, but this doesn't have to be 30 continuous minutes as it can be done in parts. Of course, if you have asthma like me, you get breathless climbing stairs or bending to use a dustpan and brush. The point I'm trying to make is that as long as you are INCREASING the amount of physical activity you do, this will benefit your diabetes.

FACT: Asthma inhalers (Ventolin, also known as Salbutamol) stimulate the pancreas to produce insulin.

Exercise is basically movement and it does not have to be a sporting activity that you specifically make time to do. How much glucose you burn off depends on the length of time you do the activity for and how much movement is involved. Housework involves some good glucose-burning activities and, while I can't tell you how many BG points you'll go down if you do them, I can tell you the calories you will burn (a calorie is a measurement of heat which is why you get hot when you are physically active – because you are burning calories as well as glucose). If the activity burns a lot of calories quickly, it also burns a lot of glucose. The following table shows how long you have to do various housework activities to burn 100 calories.

Household activity	Time to burn 100 calories
Digging the garden	12 minutes
Shoveling snow	15 minutes
Weeding the garden	18 minutes
Painting the house	18 minutes
Washing the car	20 minutes
Mowing the lawn	20 minutes
Mopping the floor	20 minutes
Vacuuming	22 minutes
Raking leaves	23 minutes
Playing with your children/Carrying a child	24 minutes
Cleaning the house	25 minutes
Shopping	25 minutes
Walking a dog	26 minutes
Pushing a pram	35 minutes
Ironing	50 minutes
Washing dishes	50 minutes

The NHS 'Preparing for DESMOND' pamphlet suggests that you assess how active you are by answering TRUE or FALSE to the following questions:

- I do some activity in my home on most days (housework; gardening, etc.)
- I try to be moderately active for 30 minutes most days.
- I always walk instead of driving if I can.
- I'm very active as part of my job/daily routine.

If you didn't do as well as you thought, perhaps this has helped to show that you could be more physically active and hopefully the list above has made you realise how.

THINKING ABOUT YOUR FOOD CHOICES

We've already talked about calories and controlling your weight but as with physical activity, you may not realise what you're actually eating until you WRITE IT DOWN. Keep a food diary before you go on your DESMOND course. Be honest as you don't have to share it with anyone else. This method really does help you see where your calories are coming from – a couple of biscuits with every cup of tea, for example, might mean an extra 300 calories a day that you don't really notice you're eating because they're not main meals. Just be aware of what you're eating and why – we often eat through boredom or because we want to cheer ourselves up. Add how you feel to your diary entry (i.e., family-sized bag of crisps because I was fed up). This is a good way of controlling your food choices a little better because you become AWARE of eating when you're not hungry.

Looking at what you eat will help the DESMOND sessions to help you. WRITE DOWN the answers to these questions:

- Do you eat the same sorts of foods each day?
- What do you usually have for breakfast?
- What do you normally have for lunch?
- What are you eating for your main meal each day?
- Do you eat supper? If so, what do you tend to have?
- What do you eat as a snack?

Look at the answers you've given and go back to when we looked at the fat and calorie contents of foods. Ask yourself, what changes do you think you could make to your diet to improve your diabetes control? You will be able to talk about making these changes on the

DESMOND course.

BEING AWARE OF YOUR MOODS

As we've already seen, BG control is hugely affected by your emotions and how you feel – feeling depressed and down increases BG while, if you have a good day, your BG can reflect this by being well-controlled. This is another aspect of the DESMOND course that you'll be able to discuss to get more support for living with and managing your diabetes. It's common to find it hard to accept the diagnosis of diabetes and you may want to also write your moods in your food and activity diary as they are related – as I've mentioned, we can eat for comfort when we're depressed and often only do what's absolutely necessary in terms of physical activity (gardening or decorating the house will not be at the top of your list if you feel fed-up). Make a note of things like:

- When something has really bothered you.
- If you feel miserable, even if your friends and family try to cheer you up.
- If you feel your self-esteem is really low (I'm stupid; I'm not as good as she is; etc.)
- When your mind wanders and you dwell on negative thoughts.
- If you feel depressed.
- If you have little interest in food and lose your appetite.
- When everything seems too much trouble.
- If you can't sleep and find yourself worrying.
- If you feel very emotional.
- If you feel unhappy, isolated and lonely.

- When you have no energy to do anything.
- When you feel happy and you think your life is going well.

The answers you give can show you how well you are coping with your diagnosis and living with your diabetes. If you feel sad and low much of the time go and see your doctor who will be able to help and provide support. Your notes on food, activity and mood will not only help you recognise patterns of behaviour in your life; they are also points to discus with the DESMOND course trainers.

REVERSING TYPE 2 DIABETES

'There are barriers to health, but the barrier should not be you'

Type 2 diabetes is thought to happen in 90% of cases because the person eats a high fat, high carbohydrate diet and takes little of no exercise. Some people with Type 2 have actually been on the receiving end of stigma where other people have blamed them and said that they have brought this on themselves. Because of the way other people view them, some people with Type 2 have stated that they feel they are blamed by health professionals and misunderstood by those with Type 1 diabetes whose condition is due to autoimmune destruction, rather than being lifestyle-related:

> Case Study
>
> Abdul Yusef was once at a diabetes clinic where a woman actually started shouting at him, saying there was nothing she could do about her Type 1 diabetes and that he was lucky because all he had to do was lose weight to get rid of his Type 2.

> Case Study
>
> Amanda Farah had been told several times by nurses, doctors and dieticians that her Type 2 diabetes was all in her own hands, that she had made herself like that because she had no self-control or motivation to exercise, and that she didn't care about her body and what she ate.

Can changing what I eat and how I exercise actually reverse Type 2 diabetes?

In recent years the number of people developing Type 2 diabetes in the United Kingdom has soared by 65% so that 3.5 million are now living with the condition. The current Type 2 diabetes epidemic (for most people, but not all) is caused by physical inactivity and obesity. The problem is now so great that health professionals in the UK cannot keep up with the number of new diagnoses. As we have just seen, the aim of the DESMOND course is to help people with Type 2 diabetes manage their condition as well as they can. Once you have the information, education and support provided by the DESMOND course you are equipped to then go forward and improve your BG control.

FACT: Dieting alone will not reverse your Type 2 – this can only be done with a complete change in your lifestyle.

Case Study

Molly Khan was 15 stone and was told she had Type 2 diabetes. This news really worried her as her mother had always had lots of problems with her own Type 2 and Molly didn't want the same. She read about a lifestyle change programme in the United States involving a low-calorie, low-fat diet with moderate exercise each day. This was supervised by health professionals and the people taking part successfully lost weight and reversed their diabetes after following the programme for 4 months. They were told that they needed to continue to lose weight until they reached a normal body mass index. Once they had reversed their diabetes and achieved a normal body weight they continued a healthy eating and exercise plan as part of their new lifestyle. A couple of people went back to their old ways of eating high fat, high carbohydrate foods and doing little or no exercise and their diabetes returned. Molly realised she needed to make a complete change to her lifestyle, consulted her GP and, after six months of determined effort, she had lost 46 pounds and her Type 2 diabetes was gone. Molly has stuck to her new lifestyle plan and is determined to never have Type 2 diabetes again.

HOW LOW ARE LOW-CARBOHTDRATE AND LOW-FAT DIETS?

Research shows that people with Type 2 diabetes who adopted a low-carbohydrate diet of less than 20g a day (the equivalent of a small apple) for six months but without any calorie restrictions for protein and fat, achieved reduced blood glucose levels and improved HbA1c results. Because carbohydrates (starch) converts to glucose in the body, low carbohydrate diets help prevent any rise in blood glucose levels. Cutting out or strictly reducing the amount of carbohydrate eaten reduces or avoids the need to take glucose-reducing medication. Lifestyle change CAN reverse Type 2 diabetes if you are very motivated to achieve this goal but YOU MUST talk to your diabetes consultant before cutting down on carbohydrates as your diabetes medication will need to be altered.

FACT: Eating a low-carbohydrate diet is not the same as a low-calorie diet. Low-carbohydrate diets allow a normal amount of fat to be eaten, meaning they are not low-calorie.

You may be advised to lose weight quickly so that you can undergo surgery (such as joint replacement) and a very low calorie diet of less than 800 calories a day may be suggested. You will only be allowed to stay on such a low-calorie diet for 12 weeks because vitamin and mineral deficiency can develop – your weight loss and general health will be supervised during this time. If you have chronic complications such as reduced liver or kidney function, cardiac impairment, disordered eating or psychological health problems, a restricted diet may not be suitable for you.

Weight-loss surgery

Weight-loss surgery, such as fitting a gastric band, has been suggested as the way to effectively tackle Type 2 diabetes in the population because it costs so much to treat the condition. Surgery may be the best option for someone who is morbidly obese (defined as a Body Mass Index of 45 and above) as low-carbohydrate and low-calorie diets may not be suitable. Keeping motivation high for losing weight is a major problem for people with Type 2 diabetes, but finding out WHY people overeat can be cheaper for the NHS than surgery:

Case Study

Suzanne Ryan had always had a weight problem and when she was 42, she developed Type 2 diabetes. With the help of a dietician and a clinical psychologist at the hospital she discovered that she often ate for comfort – it was a vicious circle because then Suzanne was unhappy because she was fat. Suzanne realised she was often just eating for the sake of it and not because she was hungry. By changing her way of thinking, Suzanne managed to lose 3 stone (42 pounds) and now her blood glucose control is normal. Her diabetes consultant has said that if she keeps the weight off, she will continue to have normal BG readings – she no longer needs to take diabetes medication.

Case Study

Dave Norris developed Type 2 diabetes when he was 35 because he viewed food as a comfort. Dave was adopted and in care homes for most of his childhood. He had never connected this with why he enjoyed his food so much. Dave paid to see a counsellor for three months and It clicked into place and made sense. Every time Dave thought about eating junk food he reminded himself of what he'd discussed with his counsellor. Dave's Type 2 diabetes control is now much better and his consultant is hoping Dave can come off Metformin completely in the near future.

FACT: Excess body fat interferes with how insulin works in body cells, causing insulin resistance and raised BG levels. Weight loss means that an amount of fat is removed from the body so insulin is able to work normally, improving BG control.

So, an improved diet and regular cardiovascular exercise has the potential to reverse Type 2 diabetes without the potentially dangerous side-effects of surgery. BUT this lifestyle change must be tailored to your specific needs by appropriately trained health professionals providing you with ongoing assistance and encouragement. As with weight loss surgery, diet and exercise is not a quick fix solution and the changes made must become permanent. This means you must be VERY motivated to succeed so you can achieve the health benefits.

Obesity is a significant risk factor for the development of many health conditions including heart disease, Type 2 diabetes, high blood pressure (*hypertension*), abnormal blood fats, such as high cholesterol, stroke, fatty deposits in the arteries (*atheroscleroisis*), and some types of cancer. Obesity is not only a risk factor for serious physical disease; it also leads to psychological conditions such as depression, disordered eating and a reduced quality of life, with complications increasing with the duration of obesity.

FACT: More than a quarter of UK adults are now classed as obese and a further 42% of men and 33% of women are overweight.

It is thought that 1.4 million morbidly obese people (with a BMI above 35) could benefit from weight loss surgery, potentially reversing 40,000 cases of Type 2 diabetes and 5,000 cases of heart disease (17 billion pounds is spent by the NHS on obesity-related conditions every year). A weight loss of 5–10% hugely improves conditions like Type 2 diabetes and heart disease that are made worse by excess body fat. As we have seen, weight loss with diet and exercise can't be achieved by people who are morbidly obese, so surgery is considered because the need to lose weight and improve Type 2 diabetes and heart disease outweighs the risks that come with this type of operation.

FACT: Having a gastric band fitted to drastically reduce the size of the stomach is not an easy option and it is not a quick fix. Significant changes to diet and exercise behaviour and lifestyle must be made so the surgery is successful.

Case Study:

Dee Vanson-Luis had a gastric band fitted to reduce the size of her stomach but she didn't receive the support to motivate her to make it work. She stuck to the diet after her surgery, eating very small meals for about a month. Then she started to cheat – having ice cream and full-fat coffees – so she actually put the 10 pounds she'd lost after having the band fitted, plus a bit more, back on again. Dee had to eventually confess to her doctor what she'd been doing and he threatened to remove the band if she wasn't going to use it properly. She felt so guilty and ashamed that it forced her to take control.

HOW WEIGHT-LOSS SURGERY WORKS

Weight-loss surgery works by severely restricting the amount of food that can be eaten by reducing the size of the stomach so less nutrients are absorbed. The stomach is re-shaped by having around 80% of it removed. There are two basic types of surgery: **restrictive surgeries and reduced absorption/restrictive surgeries.** Restrictive surgery work by physically making the size of the stomach much smaller to slow down digestion to give a feeling of fullness for longer with less food. Reduced-absorption combined with restrictive surgery involves physically removing a portion of the digestive tract to restrict the number of calories that can be absorbed by the body.

The insertion of an adjustable gastric band (also known as **lap band surgery**) is one example of restrictive surgery. This involves placing a synthetic band around the upper portion of the stomach to form a small pouch to significantly reduce the amount of food and calories that can be eaten. The size of the pouch can be altered by the surgeon by inflating or deflating the band through a port beneath the skin on the abdomen. The band can be removed at any time. Other procedures create a 'sleeve' where a small portion of the stomach is sectioned off so that it takes less food to become full, and surgery can reduce the size of the stomach and intestine to limit food and calories absorbed.

FACT: Severe vitamin deficiency can happen after having weight-loss surgery.

Reversing Type 2 diabetes with surgery

The reversal of Type 2 diabetes with surgery was first seen more than 10 years ago, although certain methods are better than others.

These methods have been successful in returning BG, insulin production and HbA1c to normal in 80–100% of morbidly obese people with Type 2 diabetes. Research shows that normal BG and insulin levels happen within days after surgery, despite the fact that there's been little or no weight loss. This means that weight loss is not the only reason insulin works better as without weight loss its action is still being increased. It is possible that the results are due to the combination of smaller meals, reduced absorption of nutrients, and a change in the gastrointestinal (GI) tract affecting how the body uses glucose.

FACT: Because of the ability of weight loss-surgery to reverse Type 2 diabetes, this will help develop new treatments for both Type 2 and obesity in the future.

Research shows that the successful reversal of Type 2 diabetes with surgery means:
- The discontinuation of BG-lowering medication.
- The achievement of normal BG levels in up to 86.6% of people.
- 80% of people become diabetes-free after their surgery.
- Normal levels of insulin are produced.
- Average weight loss is 97 pounds.
- Risk of death from obesity and Type 2 diabetes is significantly less after surgery.

FACT: People who have had Type 2 for less than 5 years and who have controlled their condition with diet achieve the best BG control after weight-loss surgery.

Possible complications following weight-loss surgery

Unfortunately, weight-loss surgery is associated with some complications depending on the type of procedure. The simpler restrictive procedures like gastric banding rarely affect the function of the bowel, so there's less risk of vitamin deficiency unless there is repeated sickness. Stomach acid can erode the synthetic band, causing abdominal pain and reduced weight loss. Sometimes the band may be over-filled by the consultant so that it slips down the stomach, making a bigger pouch for food so there is no weight loss or weight gain.

Surgery designed to reduce the absorption of nutrients is a serious procedure. There may be problems in the first few months after surgery such as:

- Poor wound healing (a particular difficulty in people with diabetes).
- Incision hernias (pushing part of the digestive tract out of its normal position) after bypass and re-joining parts of the small bowel to reduce the absorption of nutrients.
- Obstruction of the small bowel in 2.1% of cases.
- Narrowing of the small bowel in 0.7 percent of surgeries.
- Gastrointestinal bleeding in 0.6 percent of people.
- Leakage of the contents of the small bowel at the incision site in 1.2% of cases.
- Artery blockage by a blood clot (pulmonary embolus) in 1% of surgeries.
- Pneumonia in 0.1–0.3% of people following gastric bypass surgery.

There are other longer-terms complications following gastro-intestinal surgery such as:

- Lack of protein absorption causing swelling of the lower limbs and a feeling of weakness.

- Calcium, iron and vitamin deficiencies. (There must be good nutrition in the small portion sizes eaten, plus vitamin supplementation).

- Prolonged vomiting, the growth of scar tissue causing narrowing, and/or poor intestinal absorption of nutrients.

Case Study

Teresa Bull had a gastric band fitted and was told, to her delight, that she no longer had Type 2 diabetes. She frequently had heartburn and had been vomiting regularly as a complication of her surgery and six months later, Teresa developed nerve and circulatory problems due to lack of vitamin B1. She had mild peripheral neuropathy affecting the nerves in her feet because of her high BG levels when she had diabetes, but it became much worse after her weight loss surgery. Blood tests showed severe vitamin deficiencies, including iron, vitamin D and calcium, making her feel tired and weak, with muscle pain. Teresa also found she was often constipated because much less food was passing through, and she developed gallstones. She was prescribed high doses of vitamins to correct her deficiencies and laxatives to help her constipation. Despite all the side effects she experienced, Teresa feels it was worth having the surgery because she has lost 30 pounds in weight and no longer takes BG-lowering medication.

FACT: Research shows a 92% reduction in deaths from Type 2 diabetes because of weight-loss surgery.

For people recently diagnosed with Type 2 diabetes in the UK, the Department of Health agrees that weight-loss surgery to reverse the condition is an excellent way to prevent diabetic complications. This is because the cost of the surgery is outweighed by the prevention of complications and not having to treat them. Although complications can be improved with tighter or normal BG results, the damage is done and this can't be reversed:

> Case Study
>
> Patty Deane paid to have weight loss surgery two years ago. She used to take insulin for her Type 2 diabetes and, almost as soon as she'd had the operation, she didn't have to inject any more, even though Patty hadn't actually lost much weight. Unfortunately, she'd already developed eye (retinopathy) and nerve (neuropathy) complications that have not improved or gone away, despite the fact Patty's BG is now normal and so is her HbA1c.

FACT: Having a BMI of 35 and above reduces life-expectancy by 10 years.

> Case Study
>
> Dev Patel was advised to have surgery to lose weight and help his diabetes. It sounded like a great idea because Dev had always struggled with his weight and health. Although the risks were explained to him, it didn't really seem real because Dev didn't know what he'd be facing – a chance of dying just didn't seem real when he was sitting in the consultant's office. Dev just wanted to lose weight and feel better. He had problems after the operation and was very ill, needing a long stay in hospital. Dev felt that if he'd known he would experience these problems he would still have gone ahead with the surgery, but he didn't know how hard it would be to go without the pleasure of food as it's part of every occasion in life. Dev misses that, even though his diabetes has now gone because he lost just over five stones.

HOW MUCH WEIGHT WOULD I LOSE?

There is an average 47.5% loss in body weight for people who have a gastric band fitted and 61.6% of total bodyweight for those who undergo gastric bypass surgery. Weight loss tends to stabilise at around two years following surgery, and there can even be some weight gain by the third year. Perhaps more important than weight loss is the significant reversal of various weight-related health conditions. We have seen that Type 2 diabetes can successfully be treated with surgery, even before there is any great weight loss. *Metabolic syndrome* (a collection of conditions that accompany Type 2 diabetes) can also be reversed with weight loss surgery so that an early death, with its associated cardiac risk factors, can be avoided.

HOW WILL I ADJUST TO EATING MUCH LESS?

As we have seen, weight loss surgery is an extremely successful way of treating obesity, and reversing Type 2 diabetes to delay and stabilise the chronic and life-threatening complications of the disease. So, the surgery is great for improving physical health, but what about the effect on mental health because the person has to live a life of forced change which they may not be fully prepared for, despite psychological counselling?

A lot has been written about the physical complications of weight-loss surgery, but not so much about the psychological effects BEFORE and AFTER surgery. It is known that:

- Morbidly obese people experience mood disorders, anxiety and low self-esteem and are five times more likely to have suffered from major depression in the previous five years when compared with average weight individuals.

- Depression is common among morbidly obese individuals. One major factor is body dissatisfaction and this is especially the case for women, thought to be due to pressure to conform to images we see in the media.
- There is a stigma attached to obesity, leading to prejudice and discrimination which causes or worsens depression.
- Depressive symptoms are intensified by yo-yo dieting where weight loss attempts fail, increasing feelings of hopelessness and low self-esteem.
- Perhaps contributing to the complex decision to go ahead with weight-loss surgery, depressive symptoms due to the factors of body image, low self-esteem and stigma are reported by 20–30% of people at the time of their operation, with 50% saying they have a life-long history of depression.

Psychological health is closely associated with further weight gain in obese individuals and people having weight-loss surgery are more likely to suffer psychological distress compared with obese patients who don't have surgery. The trigger for some people to seek out this type of surgery (rather than it being advised by a doctor) is usually a traumatic or distressing event, such as the death of a loved one. Poor psychological health is also associated with Type 2 diabetes and obesity. As we have already seen, the impact of living with multiple health problems such as diabetes-related heart disease, blindness, kidney disease, and/or nerve pain (to name but a few consequences of diabetes complications) takes a massive toll on the individual physically and mentally.

WHO CAN HAVE WEIGHT-LOSS SURGERY?

To be eligible for this type of procedure you must have been unable to lose weight with diet and exercise and have a BMI of above 35 if you have Type 2 diabetes. Because weight-loss surgery enforces extreme dietary change it is expected that the person will adopt lifestyle change regarding their eating and exercise habits. The selection of suitable candidates for weight loss surgery involves an in-depth assessment of medical, psychological and social issues and measures are taken to assess the potential psychological impact of surgery. It is known that AFTER surgery there is:

- An improvement in depressive symptoms for 2–4 years, higher self-esteem, health-related quality of life, and a more positive body image.
- A good adaptation to behaviour change and people have reported a substantial decrease in depression and anxiety in the year following the procedure compared to obese individuals who underwent diet and exercise counselling.
- Particular improvement of depression and anxiety.

Despite the stunning success rate of weight-loss surgery in reversing obesity-related health conditions and improving overall physical and mental health, there are still a minority of people who don't feel that weight loss surgery has been a positive experience. Some find they don't have any long-term health gains or benefit following weight loss surgery. This may be because these people had unrealistic expectation of a dramatic change in their life following their surgery, setting themselves up for disappointment. This has a negative effect on mental health when expectations don't happen, even when a large amount of weight is lost:

Case Study

Laura Swain was 33 when she paid to have weight-loss surgery to reverse her Type 2 diabetes. She felt she had been stupid in expecting life to be different after she went through the surgery and lost weight. Laura had imagined that she'd be more popular, that she'd be invited out to parties and that she would be 'the life and soul'. Laura thought being thin would change everything. In reality her life hasn't changed at all – it's exactly the same except she's thinner. She still has the same life with the same problems – Laura's elderly mother, her kids, a lack of support from people. While she admits she has more confidence now to move to another job or house to make a better life, she feels she was expecting too much from the surgery and she says she's just as miserable. She'd been blaming her weight for problems in her life and has now realised that she can't do this anymore, so she is gradually accepting this.

SUPPORT FOR MAKING SURGERY WORK

After weight-loss surgery it is important to receive support and regular contact with health professionals. It is known that after the first year as clinic appointments (where people receive encouragement from health professionals) become less and less, the symptoms of depression can increase because the person feels they are on their own.

DOES WEIGHT-LOSS SURGERY INCREASE SELF-CONFIDENCE?

The person's view of how they appear to others after weight-loss surgery influences their sense of self-confidence, attractiveness and body image. This is unique to each person and this, in turn, enhances the individual's personality. Because weight-loss surgery can change body shape dramatically it is associated with increased self-esteem, self-confidence, and personality because of an improved body image and weight loss satisfaction. However, because the skin stretches with stored body fat it may not spring back again when weight is lost because our ability to do this decreases as we get older. This may cause significant distress:

Case Study

Joe England was 28 when he lost 10 stones (140 pounds) by having a gastric band fitted, exercising for 30 minutes every day and cutting out sweet and fatty foods. After his dramatic weight loss his Type 2 diabetes disappeared but his new 12-stone shape had folds of skin hanging from his arms, legs and chest. He hadn't expected to have so much skin hanging everywhere and he viewed this skin as ugly. Despite this, Joe was pleased with his overall appearance and he felt good about his body image. Joe has arranged to have a second operation to remove the skin on the underside of his arms and more surgery to have his legs done, a tummy tuck and bottom lift. He is prepared for the extensive scars everywhere but wishes he'd now got the body he dreamed of. He just wanted to fix the problem when he woke up after the surgery – that the fat would be gone.

CAN CHILDREN HAVE WEIGHT-LOSS SURGERY?

There are now more and more cases of children who are developing Type 2 diabetes because they eat an unhealthy diet and do little or no exercise. Increasing rates of extreme obesity in children are being reported and with this alarming trend comes not only Type 2 diabetes but also other 'adult' diseases such as *obstructive sleep apnoea* (where fat around the neck interferes with breathing during sleep); fatty liver disease, and heart disease, with severely obese adolescents being at particular risk. Obese children are also known to experience significant hostility from others; low self-esteem; body dissatisfaction; depressive symptoms; poor control of what they are eating; harmful weight control behaviours (such as *anorexia* and/or *bulimia*); and are less able to be sociable and make friends; these problems being worse in girls than boys.

FACT: Tackling the problem of childhood obesity involves the whole family as obesity is often related to poor nutrition and family understanding of portion control. Reducing calories and increasing the amount of regular exercise will benefit the whole family.

Weight-loss surgery is considered for young persons with life-threatening obesity but this is only in extreme cases where the need outweighs the risk as doctors prefer that diet, exercise and weight-loss medication are the first things tried. The success rate of weight-loss surgery in adolescents is similar to that in adults, with 40–60% of excess weight lost in the first year and upwards of 75% by the end of the second year. Weight loss surgery in young adults has the same effect as in older individuals of improving high blood pressure, insulin resistance, Type 2 diabetes and high levels of unhealthy blood fats. Psychologically, depression, anxiety and self-image are also improved following stomach-reducing procedures after as little as four months and this improvement lasts for more than four years. This shows that mental health is strongly associated with weight control.

FACT: A weight-loss surgeon must feel that the need to improve the health of a young person is greater than the risk of having surgery.

WHAT DIABETES CARE SHOULD I RECEIVE?

'Going into hospital worries me because I can't be in control of my diabetes'

You may not know it but as a person with diabetes in the UK, you are entitled to receive a certain level of care. (This will be different in countries such as the USA and Australia where healthcare is dependent on health insurance.) This level of care is laid down by UK law so if you don't get the right diabetes care you can take this matter to court. If you are anything like me you won't even question diabetes care in your area, or know what the right sort of care is. There are certain rights that you should have as standard without having to ask, such as:

- Getting most healthcare, free of charge.
- Being able to have the GP you want, although they can refuse you. If you can't find a GP in your area, your Local Authority can help. (You can change your GP when you like without giving them notice).
- The right to see your medical records. (This can be refused if it's felt that seeing them may cause you distress or if a third party is mentioned in part of the records who has said they don't want the records to be seen).
- The right to refuse treatment, unless it's covered by the Mental Health Act, 1983.
- The right for your information to be confidential within the NHS as part of your treatment.
- The right for any complaint you make against the NHS to be investigated using the NHS complaints procedure.

- Possible refund of travel costs to hospital, NHS prescription charges, NHS dental charges, NHS sight tests, glasses and contact lenses, wigs and fabric supports. Information about refunds can be found at your local Benefit Agency.

FACT: Make sure you know what you're entitled to so you get the best out of the NHS.

So, now you know your rights to general health care, what about your rights to specialist diabetes care? Recent reports in the news have highlighted patchy diabetes care across the country. To get the best out of the system you need to be prepared to work with health professionals so that you are PART of your diabetes team. After all, YOU are the most important person in this team! Knowing as much as you can about your diabetes is the key to being able to discuss your condition and getting what you need to manage it properly.

FACT: You can discuss the roles and responsibilities of your diabetes care team with your GP.

Who's who? Your diabetes care team includes:
- YOU
- Your diabetes consultant (also known as your diabetologist or endocrinologist).
- Your diabetes specialist nurse (DSN).
- Your General Practitioner (GP).
- Your Practice Nurse (at your GP surgery).
- A dietician.

- An optometrist or ophthalmologist to care for your eyes.
- A podiatrist or chiropodist to care for your feet.
- A psychologist or diabetes-trained counsellor.
- Your pharmacist.

You may see some members of your diabetes team more often than others, especially when you are first diagnosed with diabetes. As this is the time when everything is new and you are having to take in lots of information about your condition, your diabetes team should:

- Provide you with a full medical examination.
- Decide on a plan of diabetes care with you.
- Introduce you to a diabetes specialist nurse who will explain the condition, your treatment and how to use diabetes self-care equipment such as a BG testing monitor.
- Teach you how to manage your own diabetes.
- Arrange a meeting with a dietician so you can discuss what you eat and get advice on how to improve your diet to help your BG control.
- Explain the importance of a healthy diet and regular exercise.
- Explain how diabetes may affect your lifestyle in terms of issues such as work, driving a vehicle, travel and life insurance.
- Provide ongoing information and education about diabetes-related issues as necessary.
- Give you information about local diabetes support groups.

FACT: Once your diabetes is under control you will see your diabetes team at least once a year for an annual review, although you should be able to contact them for advice when you need it.

After you have met your diabetes team they should provide you with:

- Ongoing care based on a full knowledge of your needs and medical history.
- Periodically review and help you achieve your diabetes management goals.
- The opportunity to be involved in your diabetes care decisions.
- Advice before, during and after pregnancy as part of your maternity team.
- Advice about diabetes if you have carers that visit you at home.
- The opportunity to involve relatives, partners and friends in giving you support.
- The educational sessions and appointments you need.
- Information about managing your diabetes medication when you are ill.

If you take insulin you will learn

- How to inject yourself and how to store your insulin.
- How to dispose of syringes and needles.
- How to test your BG for glucose and your urine for ketones and what the results mean.

- How to recognise and treat low BG.

You will also be given insulin supplies (or a prescription for insulin) and the equipment you need to give yourself insulin and test your BG.

If your diabetes is treated with tablets you will learn:
- How to test your blood and urine for glucose and what the results mean.
- When low BG may happen and how to deal with it.

You will also be given a supply of your glucose-reducing tablets (or a prescription for them) and blood and urine testing equipment.

If your diabetes is managed by diet you will:
- Receive blood and urine glucose testing equipment and be told what the results mean.

FACT: Your first prescription will be provided by your hospital diabetes clinic. Ongoing prescriptions will need to be ordered from your GP surgery. Prescriptions of insulin, needles, BG-lowering medication, lancets and test strips are FREE with an exemption certificate (from your local health authority). BG testing meters may have to be bought.

What to expect when you see the diabetes nurse

Annual monitoring if you have Type 1 diabetes will involve having BG, blood pressure and weight measured and recording these with the result of your last HbA1c test to see if there are any changes. A urine sample will be taken to test for glucose, ketones, and protein.

If you have Type 2 diabetes, your consultation with the diabetes nurse will involve measurement of blood pressure (to check for high blood pressure) and urine to check for any kidney changes, especially if you have poor BG control. A cardiovascular function (heart and circulatory system) and diabetes complications risk assessment is also carried out, as well as measures to manage blood fats, and introducing tablets (statins) to reduce cholesterol levels if necessary. You may also be advised to take a 75mg daily dose of aspirin to prevent blood clots.

What to expect when you see your diabetes consultant

As a person will diabetes you will periodically have an appointment for a consultation with your diabetes specialist (unless you have Type 2 diabetes and receive your care from your GP practice). Even if this is the case, there are certain things that you should expect from your appointment:

- To receive regular health checks such as HbA1c blood testing for glucose levels, urine testing and foot examination.
- To be informed of changes in your condition that may lead to diabetic complications; to be advised of any changes in your care; to have test results simply explained in a way you can understand; to discuss lifestyle issues that may be affecting your BG control; to provide you with ongoing education about your diabetes; and to answer any questions you might have.
- Come prepared with a list of questions that you have written down so you can remind yourself if you get side-tracked; read as much as you can about diabetes so you are confident, informed and in a position to discuss your

condition; find out how much time you'll have with your consultant or other health professionals by asking when you check in for your appointment at reception; bring a sample of urine and your BG monitoring diary with you.

Do I have any responsibilities as a diabetes team member?

As I mentioned earlier, diabetes is a health condition where 95% of the care needed to manage it properly is down to YOU. While this is true, you can't do everything on your own and you need to work with your diabetes care team to keep your diabetes under control. They will help you to fit diabetes into your lifestyle so that you see the benefits to your health. This is because getting your diabetes care right is not easy, so your diabetes care team is there to help. As you are the person that is in charge of your diabetes you must:

- Be responsible for as much of your own day-to-day diabetes care as possible. This means finding out all you can about your condition to make the management easier.
- Include making appropriate food choices, exercise and regular BG monitoring into your diabetes self-management routine.
- Check your feet daily, or as often as you can. If you can't do it, ask someone else.
- Ask for help to manage your diabetes if and when you need it, such as when you are ill with an infection or stomach upset.
- Know who, when and where to contact the people who can help you.

- Take on the diabetes management advice you receive and ask your diabetes team for the information and advice you need. MAKE A LIST of things to ask so you don't forget.
- Go to your diabetes clinic appointments, and any others that will help you such as eye and foot care appointments.

What about if I have to go into hospital and can't be in control?

Going into hospital is always a worrying time, whether it's related to your diabetes or not. Once you are in hospital your care is shared between you and the health professionals on the ward. It can be difficult to maintain good BG control when you are not living your normal lifestyle – your BG may be much higher because you're not physically active for a period of time. You will need to increase your insulin or BG-lowering medication to cover this inactivity so your BG is as near-normal as possible – this will help you to heal more quickly, especially if you have had an operation. You should have the opportunity to discuss any concerns you have with a doctor or nurse before you are admitted to hospital, or once you are there. During your stay in hospital:

- You will receive an explanation of your medical treatment while you are in hospital.
- You will be able to inform ward staff about your dietary needs, tablets or insulin treatment.
- You will be able to inform your hospital diabetes team of your admission.
- You will be able to do your own blood and urine glucose monitoring (and insulin injections) if you are well enough.

- Your insulin (if you take it) may be given in an intravenous drip with glucose if you are not allowed to eat before an operation. Your BG control will be managed by an anaesthetist during your operation.

- Your dosage of BG-lowering medication will change and you may be put onto insulin temporarily.

- You should bring supplies of sweet foods to reverse low BG if you use insulin or sulphonylureas to treat your diabetes. Tell the nursing staff if you do have a hypo.

- Your diabetes control will be worse because you are not moving about, you are in a different environment and you may experience pain that can increase BG.

Case Study

Mark King was admitted to hospital to have a hip replacement operation. He was worried about having to hand over control of his Type 1 diabetes to health professionals who didn't know him or his routine. When he was admitted a nurse, Kay, came to find out about when Mark usually did his insulin injections and BG monitoring. Kay also explained Mark's surgical procedure and how his diabetes would be managed until he left hospital. Kay informed the hospital diabetes team of Mark's admission, told him when mealtimes were so he could give his insulin accordingly, and assured him that he would only be seen by staff fully trained in the care of patients with diabetes. Mark was advised about returning to his usual insulin treatment when he left hospital and that he would have regular check-ups when he left hospital. This personal care helped Mark to feel confident about managing his diabetes during his stay in hospital.

FACT: The staff on hospital wards are very used to helping people with diabetes so don't worry – they will be familiar with what you have to do to manage your condition.

Case Study

Shian Serei had Type 2 diabetes and a bad chest infection. Her GP arranged to admit her to hospital because she had ketones in her urine and high BG levels because of the infection. Shian was worried about going into hospital because she didn't speak English very well, but her sister spoke to Shian's diabetes nurse over the phone and she advised that Shian should take a family member who could speak English along with her when she was admitted so they could interpret for Shian and make sure she received culturally-appropriate diabetes care while she was in hospital. This gave Shian peace of mind as the worry was not helping her BG levels. Having her family members involved in her hospital diabetes care also helped Shian recover more quickly and she was able to go home a week later once her diabetes was stabilised.

FACT: If you have been waiting a long time for your hospital diabetes check-up or follow-up appointment you should contact your GP so they can chase this up for you.

HOW TO MAKE A COMPLAINT ABOUT YOUR DIABETES CARE

If you have a complaint about the NHS diabetes care you receive in the UK, you should speak to your GP and/or your diabetes team as the people providing your care because they have a complaints procedure. You will be asked to put your complaint in writing and you will be told to contact PALS (the Patient and Liaison Service) who can act as a go between as your complaint is investigated. This may take some time, but you will receive an outcome.

If the way your complaint is handled, or the reply you receive is not satisfactory to you, you can take the matter to your local Health Authority complaints office so that it can be considered by an impartial review panel. If this fails to resolve the issue you can take the matter even further to the Health Service Ombudsman so it can be investigated. Your local Community Health Council (CHC) can give you the details of how to contact the Health Service Ombudsman.

YOUNG AND OLD

'The public needs to be shown that anyone can be affected by diabetes'

Babies and small children with diabetes

FACT: Cases of Type 1 diabetes are increasing, especially in children under 5 years old, with a recent 6.3% annual increase in cases compared to an overall increase of 3.4% across all age groups.

BABIES AND TODDLERS WITH TYPE 1 DIABETES

When a baby or pre-school toddler with limited language skills becomes diabetic they obviously can't tell you that they feel unwell. If your baby has not progressed to potty training you won't be able to tell how much urine is being passed into their nappy and if your baby has diarrhoea and vomiting and/or losses weight you might think they have a tummy upset. Because of these factors it may be some time before diabetes is diagnosed and your baby could be very ill by that time. Your baby will be admitted to the paediatric intensive care unit at the hospital so that insulin treatment can begin but it is important that you DON'T BLAME YOURSELF – there is no way you could have known that your baby or toddler had undiagnosed diabetes.

When you finally have a diagnosis you will learn how to give your baby or pre-school child daily insulin and test BG. Because both are unpleasant for the child they won't be willing participants and this is something else you must come to terms with – your baby needs to have insulin and BG checks, so you are doing this for them and you must overcome the feeling that you are stressing them or hurting them. You will also learn how to feed your baby regularly with the right food to prevent low BG.

Although the emphasis is on good control of BG in diabetes, in the case of babies with the condition this is less important because the nervous system has not fully developed and therefore can't be affected by high BG levels. It is frequent HYPOGLYCAEMIA that causes damage to the developing nerves rather than high BG, so you are aiming to prevent this. The good news for babies and children is that damage from high BG levels doesn't start to happen until just before the child reaches puberty. It is important to remember that small changes in the chemical balance of a baby's system can have a big effect, so they become ill quickly. Aim to keep your baby's BG between 8.3–11.0 mmol/L.

FACT: Young people experience a *honeymoon period* after Type 1 diabetes is diagnosed where they need very little insulin to keep BG under control. Unfortunately, this doesn't last.

The honeymoon period will last longer in older children, if the symptoms of Type 1 diabetes before diagnosis were mild rather than dramatic, and if the body's attack on the insulin-producing cells of the pancreases is not sufficient to wipe out all cells as soon as they are formed. When the honeymoon period ends and the pancreas stops producing insulin again in Type 1 diabetes (up to a period of 3 years), BG will begin to rise again and the diabetes team looking after your child will work out how much insulin they need to control your child's condition. You will then be taught to:

- Recognise the signs of high and low BG and diabetic ketoacidosis (sickness and vomiting, rapid breathing, sleepiness/drowsy, weakness).
- Give insulin (short acting fits better with children's irregular eating habits).
- Test BG and urine ketone levels.
- Treat low BG with glucose or a Glucagen injection kit.
- Feed a baby or child who has diabetes.
- React when your child is ill with an illness other than diabetes.

Because your child can't carry out its own diabetes self-care, managing your baby or toddler's diabetes is very demanding. This also causes anxiety when you have to hand over your child's care to someone else for a time. Toddlers learn to become more independent as they approach the time they go to school. This can be difficult because your child needs you to continue to carry out their diabetes management for them. The responsibilities of caring for a diabetic child mean you will have little time to do anything else.

FACT: It is common for the siblings of a diabetic child to become jealous of the extra attention paid to their brother or sister, even if they understand that you are doing things like injections and blood tests.

TYPE 2 DIABETES

Although Type 2 diabetes is traditionally a condition seen in middle age, children as young as 7 years of age are now also developing this disease. Some children are more at risk than others of having insulin resistance (when insulin can't work properly), and then Type

2 diabetes as a result. The reasons for insulin resistance developing in the very young are:

- Increased weight above normal childhood weight gain.
- A family history of insulin resistance and Type 2 diabetes.
- Being from a racial minority group such as South-East Asians, Native Americans, Pacific Islanders, and African Americans.
- Low birth weight has been a factor in historical records, but not current records.

The reason for identifying babies and children with insulin resistance is to be able to suggest the family make lifestyle changes before the young person develops Type 2 diabetes. As in adults who make changes to their diet and increase their physical activity, cases of insulin resistance in the young can be reversed and Type 2 can be avoided or delayed.

FACT: Children with any of the above risk factors should have their fasting BG measured and followed up regularly by their GP or Practice Nurse.

Care of children with diabetes at school

Once your child starts school, having diabetes becomes slightly easier as they can let you know how they feel, so hypos are easier to detect, but BG control can become more difficult as your child is not in your care during the day. Because there are so many more children getting Type 1 diabetes now there are more who have to face the challenges of having this condition in school. The Department of Health says that children and young people spend a quarter of their daily lives at school and currently, one in 550 school children has Type 1 diabetes and 85% of these has a HbA1c of above 7.7%. This means that their diabetes IS NOT well controlled (although high BG levels don't start to do damage until the child reaches puberty). Children usually spend a third of their day in school or nursery care, so the staff there MUST be told and understand the importance of managing your child's diabetes.

FACT: Diabetes health professionals can educate and train school staff so they can support your child and manage their condition while they are away from home.

In an attempt to gain good BG control with insulin treatments, multiple daily injections (MDI) and insulin pump therapy are used to manage Type 1 diabetes in children as soon as it is diagnosed. This is because these treatments are flexible in that dosages can be adjusted for different foods and so that BG results are within normal range. The hospital diabetes team will involve you and your child in deciding on the best choice of insulin treatment and will give you and your child the necessary information and education to use it correctly.

As the name suggests, multiple daily injections of insulin mean these need to be done throughout the day to keep BG levels as normal as possible, avoiding high and low glucose swings. Your child will need an injection of insulin at lunchtime and most children from 9–16 years old will do this themselves but if not, either the parent or a member of school staff has to give the injection as needles have to be supervised closely in school for health and safety reasons (the same goes for BG testing with lancets).

Some parents are unable to come into school at lunchtime to do their child's injection so it is very important that the school and the member of staff (usually a school nurse) knows exactly what needs to be done and when. It is generally thought that children of 11 years of age who have had Type 1 diabetes for some time can be independent and inject their own insulin at school (with the nurse present).

An insulin pump is attached to the body 24/7 and if your child uses this way of delivering their insulin, they will go to see the school nurse at lunchtime to have their BG monitored and to get their insulin dose before they eat. Insulin pumps have a lock function to stop the pump giving a bolus (dose) of insulin unless it is specifically needed. This prevents children from pressing buttons on the pump and giving unnecessary insulin that could cause low BG.

Pumps can also work with a glucose sensor to warn of high and low glucose levels if your child has difficult to manage (brittle) Type 1. This means that all of your child's teachers need to be aware that the pump alarm may sound during lessons and that your child will need to go to the school nurse so that glucose, or a bolus of insulin if BG is very high, can be given. (But if it's a hypo, the child should be treated for low BG WHERE THEY ARE – not sent anywhere else – especially if the reading shows a very low BG)

FACT: School staff are under a common duty-of-care law to make sure children with diabetes are healthy and safe. This law covers administering medication as well as action in an emergency including the treatment of hypoglycaemia.

The ideal situation for a child with diabetes is for BG results at school to be as good as when they are at home. Schools and Local Education Authorities (LEAS) are obliged NOT to treat children with diabetes less favourably than those without diabetes unless they can provide a valid reason. This means that schools CAN'T STATE that they will not administer medication of any kind or insist that parents must come into school to do this for their child. It can be very difficult and worrying for a parent to hand over the care of their child to the school during the day, and for this to be right the school MUST be fully aware of their role in your child's daily diabetes management:

Case Study

Susan Parker's son, Ben, was diagnosed with Type 1 diabetes when he was 6 years old. Susan worked full-time but came into the school to give Ben his insulin every lunchtime for three months. She then made it clear to the school that it was their responsibility to manage Ben's diabetes during the day while he was in their care. Susan spoke with Ben's Children's Diabetes Nurse Specialist (CDNS) and they both visited Ben's school to discuss the staff's responsibilities in administering Ben's necessary injections. Once the school was clear on their role in Ben's diabetes care, Susan found there were no more problems.

Below is a list of knowledge and skills that your child's school should have to support a child with diabetes of up to 11 years of age:

- Awareness to test BG if a child says they feel unwell as symptoms of low BG can be confused with high BG. It is important to test BG BEFORE any glucose or insulin is given.

- Ability to recognise the symptoms of low BG as young children may not be able to do this, especially if they are playing or concentrating in class.
- Ability to treat low BG of less than 4 mmol/L as young children may not be able to do this themselves, especially if they are disorientated by low BG. The child SHOULD NOT be sent anywhere else to treat their hypo.
- Approachable by the child and able to act quickly on the child's behalf as young children may not feel confident and able to approach an adult in authority.
- Ability to supervise and support BG testing as young children need to be reminded to wash their hands and may need help with the testing process, especially when interpreting the results.
- Ability to supervise the child giving insulin via a pen or pump.
- Ability to help the child calculate the carbohydrate content of meals and awareness that a child may eat more if they share food with others, or less if they drop food or don't want to eat part of their meal.
- Ability to plan ahead for exercise so that glucose is taken or is available as children may forget or be distracted.
- IF THE CHILD USES PUMP THERAPY, the ability to help the child with numeracy skills when calculating insulin or programming an insulin pump where the position of the decimal point on insulin delivery is crucial, i.e. the difference between 10.0 units and 1.0 unit of insulin.
- It is especially important that the adult knows how to SUSPEND insulin delivery on the pump when the child has low BG (although there is an auto-suspend function on some

models) as their own ability may be impaired, and when to RESUME insulin delivery once BG has returned to normal.

- Ability to recognise pump equipment problems such as NO DELIVERY of insulin, understanding the meanings of pump alarms, and knowing who to contact.

FACT: Schools do not currently do testing of children's urine for ketone in cases of illness and when there is very high BG, so parents have to come into school to do this.

FACT: Schools do not currently support the use of Glucagen injection kits in cases of severe hypoglycaemia and will phone the emergency services to do this.

Case Study

Peter Davis received a phone call at work to say that his 10-year-old daughter, Lisa, was having a bad hypo. She'd been running around the playground with her friends and collapsed during an afternoon class, shaking and sweating. Lisa's teacher called an ambulance because she'd been told this was an emergency situation. Peter Davis quickly left work, stopped off at home to grab a Glucagen injection kit, and rushed to Lisa's school. When Peter arrived he found Lisa had been taken to the school nurse's room because the other children were frightened of the way she was acting. The nurse and the ambulance man were panicking because the paramedic said he was not trained to give Glucagen. Peter was very angry and pushed past them to give Lisa the injection he had bought from home before she dropped into unconsciousness. Peter did a BG test on Lisa and found she was 2.5mmol/L. After ten minutes, Lisa became more coherent and her next BG was 5.0 mmol/L. Peter took Lisa home, although she was fine after her severely low BG had been treated in the same way Peter would do at home. Peter warns other parents to always take a Glucagen injection kit along to the school if they phone to say a diabetic child is ill.

FACT: As you begin to tighten your child's BG control as they grow older there is more chance of low BG, especially during the night.

HYPO-BUSTING TIPS

When you tighten your child's BG control there is less glucose in the blood so hypos can happen more often. This is often the case at bedtime, after an evening meal has been digested but there is still working insulin in the bloodstream. When your child goes to bed, make sure that you:

- Give them a bedtime snack, such as a couple of plain biscuits.
- Check your child's BG before they go to sleep.
- Ask your child if they have experienced symptoms of low BG during the night, such as nightmares or headaches. Do an occasional BG test at 3 a.m.
- Know if your child hasn't eaten all of their meal.
- Give your child extra carbohydrate to eat before exercising.
- Tell your child's school who to contact in an emergency.

FACT: Frequent hypoglycaemia in children DOES NOT damage a child's brain.

It is helpful to take your child to the supermarket so they can learn about food labels, foods that are high in calories, fats and carbohydrates, especially if you have been told by your child's diabetes consultant that they need to lose some weight. When I was first diagnosed at age 10, although I was thin because I wasn't 'allowed' to eat certain foods, this made them very desirable. I would take a detour to the shops on my way to school and visit the bakery, or buy crisps and chocolate and in my 10-year old mind, I thought I was getting back at the doctors, not realising that I was on a restricted diet for a reason.

Diabetes in this day and age is completely different because of Dosage Adjustment For Normal Eating (DAFNE) so children don't have to miss out on the occasional treat, especially if they have low BG or are about to exercise. This makes it easier if you also have other non-diabetic children who don't have to watch their diet. Make sure that you NEVER use food with high calories like cake or sweets as a reward so that your child knows it's better to eat a banana for carbohydrate than crisps.

DIET & EXERCISE

- Nutritional needs for children change constantly as they grow. It's important to speak to the dietician in your child's diabetes team when they have a growth spurt because they will be eating much more food for cell growth.
- Children can be very physically active, especially when playing with friends. Make sure they are aware that running around can cause hypos.
- Help your child make the right food choices and let them decide that what they want to eat that fits with those choice. They are more likely to eat their meals if they've had some input and they like what they've chosen.
- Children need a certain level of fat in their diet as they grow and their body develops so, for this reason, children under two years old (or those who won't eat properly) should be

given full-fat milk, yoghurt and cheese rather than low-fat varieties.

- High-fibre foods are not a good choice for young children so give them unsweetened cereals, rice, pasta, potatoes, and fruit instead.

- School meals can be healthy options like jacket potatoes with baked beans rather than chips. Make sure your child knows how to make healthy food choices and why this is important for their health.

- It's NORMAL to worry about what your child eats and how much physical activity they do when they're at school or visiting a friend's house. The hospital dietician can help here by giving suggestions.

FACT: Buying 'diabetic' chocolate, sweets, cakes or ice cream is a waste of time. They are usually more expensive, don't always taste nice, and still contain sugar or a sweetener that can cause diahorrea. It's better for your child to eat normal foods in measured amounts and have the insulin dosage necessary for the carbohydrate content.

Teenagers with Type 1 diabetes

Most cases of Type 1 diabetes happen during the teenage years. If it was diagnosed earlier than this, your child will have been afforded some protection from the risk of complications, but once they reach 13 years of age, BG must be controlled to prevent this. Diabetes self-management is difficult at any age, but being a teenager makes this even more challenging. Teenagers don't think of long-term complications of diabetes – I certainly didn't – and, like me, they can be unwilling to test their BG regularly. There are lots of issues for this age group that make managing diabetes difficult, such as:

- Hormonal changes during puberty increasing BG because of insulin resistance.
- Increased risk of ketosis in association with high BG.
- A desire to be independent.
- Trying to remain and identify within the group-thinking of friends (peer pressure).
- Resisting authority.
- Changing from child (paediatric) to adult diabetes clinics for their care.

Your child's desire to become independent is probably one of the biggest challenges you will face as a parent. Although this might seem like a good idea, especially in letting them take control of their own diabetes, you should hold on to the reins of diabetes control for your child for several reasons:

- Clear rules from you that can be followed mean better BG control for your child.
- Your child may want to act like friends do when they are around, meaning injections and BG tests are missed.
- Teenagers may still be unable or unwilling to interpret BG results and act upon them.
- Weight issues, especially in girls, may start to trouble your child. There is a condition called *diabulimia* (thought to affect one-third of women and young girls with Type 1 diabetes) where insulin is reduced or completely omitted to induce ketoacidosis and rapid weight loss. This is done very secretively and parents may not even know it's happening

repeatedly, putting the young person at risk of diabetic ketoacidosis and chronic and severe complications such as eye, nerve and kidney disease.

FACT: Diabulimia is not a condition recognised by the medical profession. Although it is deliberate diabetes miss-management it is classed as an eating disorder.

Case Study

Alissa Thomas developed Type 1 diabetes when she was 11 and soon found out that, when she was ill with diabetic ketoacidosis, she could lose about a stone (14 pounds) in a week. Alissa was admitted to hospital several times with DKA because she had repeated chest infections, and found out that DKA is due to hyperglycaemia and a lack of insulin. Instead of being extra careful about her BG levels when she had a cold or a chest infection, Alissa used this as an opportunity to lose weight, although she knew it was dangerous and could affect her sight and her heart function. As Alissa grew older she became more and more aware of her weight and body image (although she was actually underweight for her height) and she began cutting down on the amount of insulin she took so that she felt sick, had little appetite and lost weight. Alissa's parents had always thought that she'd lost weight each time she was ill, but they began to notice that she skipped meals and was losing weight when she was apparently well. They took her to her doctor and tests showed that Alissa had ketones in her urine. The doctor explained that Alissa already had early signs of retinopathy associated with continually high BG levels and that if she carried on under-dosing on her insulin, she could damage other vital organs as well. Alissa realised how much damage she was doing to her body and began looking after her diabetes properly, although she admits that it's still very tempting to try and lose weight this way if there's an important event she is attending.

FACT: DKA is a dangerous, serious acute medical condition and it is fatal in 10% of cases (especially if there's other illness to complicate DKA), so do not be tempted to reduce or omit your insulin to try and lose weight quickly.

Case Study

Drew Morris was 14 when he started being bullied about both his diabetes and his weight. Although people with Type 1 diabetes tend to be lean, Drew was slightly overweight for his height because he enjoyed eating regular pizza and Italian food with creamy sauces. When he moved house with his parents, Drew started at a new school and found he was being teased and picked on. He tried to shrug it off, but the comments really got to him and he began trying to take control of the situation by under-dosing on the amount of insulin he should have been taking. This was Drew's way of taking action, although he didn't realise how dangerous it was. He noticed that his BG tests were much higher because he had less insulin in his bloodstream and he also found that he was losing weight steadily. Drew's parents thought this was because he was attending an after-school sports club, but this wasn't true. Eventually Drew became very ill with DKA and was admitted to hospital. He underwent tests and it was discovered that he had early kidney damage related to his high BG levels over time. Drew felt guilty that he had done this to himself, especially as his mother was telling him it was such a shame that diabetes had affected him like this. Drew knew he could have prevented this damage. From that day he decided to manage his diabetes well to prevent any further kidney damage from high BG levels.

As we have seen, it can be difficult to get young people to participate in looking after their diabetes. Hospital diabetes teams (paediatric diabetes clinics) caring for teenagers with the condition now use technology to try and engage teenager in their diabetes care. Methods such as texting reminders to your child's mobile phone to test BG, and for young patients to text their blood results back to be recorded as a measure of diabetes self-management as well as estimated monthly HbA1c values have been successful. Using modern technology in this way provides easily accessible support and helps the young person to gain better control of their BG levels. This method has been successful because it breaks down barriers between the hospital diabetes clinic and the teenager with diabetes because they're willing to engage with technology to receive and send messages about their diabetes:

Case Study

Joel Pinder-King is 15 and has had Type 1 diabetes since he was 6 years old. He tends to not take it too seriously, doing the same things his friends do without making sure he has glucose with him. Joel also sometimes forgets to do his insulin injections, or takes them at the wrong times when he remembers. Joel's BG results are usually either too low or too high because of the way he manages his condition. Joel's diabetes nurse suggested he text his BG results to a web address he was given so the information can be stored and analysed and he agreed. Joel also agreed that he was happy to receive text alert reminders such as to have his insulin at certain times throughout the day. After 3 months of this Joel's diabetes control is much better. He said that the system works for him because it reminds him to test his BG and do his injections on time; stops him eating so much chocolate and he can receive clinic appointment reminders; get his diabetes-related questions answered quickly; and see that other people feel the same way about their diabetes. Joel also found out that he shouldn't inject his insulin through his clothes.

Students managing diabetes away from home

There comes a time when your child will need to be independent and you will need to pass their diabetes control fully over to them. By this time your child will have been doing their own injections and BG testing for a number of years, managing their condition and knowing what they need to do and when. BUT, if they then became

Ill, it was reassuring to know you were there. Now, if your child is leaving home for the first time to go away to college or university, they will need to become fully independent.

A 70% rise in Type 1 diabetes is predicted in young people aged 15 and above over the next few years. Very little has been written about the experiences of young adults with diabetes who leave home to go to college or university, so it's a case of trial and error. This massive change presents the challenges of juggling diabetes self-management, establishing their own identity, dealing with peer group and authority pressures, and hormonal variations which can stop insulin working as well (insulin resistance) so more insulin is needed. This upheaval may be made worse by the need for your child to transfer from paediatric to adult diabetes care at this time.

BALANCING DIABETES AND FURTHER EDUCATION

All students experience stress, but this can complicate diabetes by increasing BG levels. Being in a different environment with a different routine can also make injecting insulin several times a day, BG testing and eating on time much more difficult, but after a while the new routine will become easier and your child will get to know when they are likely to become low so they can eat some glucose tablets if they can't get any food at the time, such as if they're in class. Time may not be the only issue: your child may not want to attract attention by insisting they have to eat or inject:

Case Study

Emma Khan is 18 and has Type 1 diabetes. She's in her first year at university and has found the change very difficult because university is not as flexible as her school used to be

In letting her go out of class to test her BG or inject her insulin. Some days the lectures are 9–6 with an hour for lunch at 12 noon and on others they are 9–1 with no lunch break but the afternoon off. Emma doesn't have time to test her BG between lectures and she finds it embarrassing to make an issue of it. She has found that she has got into a routine of not testing her BG when she's with people and having less insulin to avoid hypoglycaemia, although she knows it's dangerous. She only tests her BG now when she feels sick and it affects her ability to work or concentrate.

Students often feel that they don't receive adequate support from their college/university and their diabetes team so they can manage the demands of further education and diabetes self-management.

Case Study

Paige Wells is in her second year at university but doesn't find managing her Type 1 diabetes any easier when she's away from home. Paige feels that despite the fact she has told the university about her diabetes, and her diabetes team that she's at university, she's left to manage on her own. She once told one of her tutors that she needed a break during a three-hour exam to check her BG and he replied that Paige should have made sure she could sit through the exam without interruption. On another occasion, Paige tried to organise an appointment with her new (adult) diabetes team, but they said she needed a referral from her GP who was 300 miles away in her home town. Her paediatric team also said they could no longer see her as she must transfer to the adult clinic. Paige felt stuck in the middle, abandoned with no one to help or support her. She added that this must be a common problem for young people with diabetes.

ADVERSE DIABETES MANAGEMENT STRATEGIES

Hypoglycaemia is a massive worry when you have diabetes and you are away from home when you don't feel confident you can deal with it. I recall a particularly horrible incident when I was away at a new university where no one knew me – funnily enough, attending a three-day diabetes conference, surrounded by diabetes consultants from all over the world! On the way from dropping off my stuff in my room, having crossed a rather busy road, I succumbed to a very severe and unexpected hypo with no warning signs and collapsed unconscious in some bushes. After a while I managed to stagger to the porter's lodge where I flung open the door, announced in a slurred and confused voice that the porter should phone my husband, and dropped into unconsciousness again. I was very, very lucky that the porter then phoned one of the course tutors – an expert in hypoglycaemia who came rushing over with a Glucagen injection to bring me round. To this day I shudder to think what might have happened if I'd been attending a course on flower arranging or car maintenance!

The above example is something that people who take insulin fear the most – losing control and having to rely on someone else to know what to do. I was so embarrassed and felt so ill after that incident that I phoned my husband (having refused and ambulance) and he drove 150 miles to take me home. This fear of the disabling effects of hypoglycaemia causes some people to deliberately take less insulin than they need so their BG tends to be too high rather than too low. This tactic is especially true of students who want to fit in and don't want the fuss and embarrassment of a public hypo:

Case Study

Vin Gupta says that she absolutely hates having hypos because they take away her feeling of control. She explained that it's impossible to tell everyone you have to deal with what a hypo is and how to treat it. Vin's doctor told her she had to take responsibility for her own diabetes, especially because she's away from home. Because she is continually worried, Vin finds it easier to run higher BG levels so she doesn't have a hypo, although one day she knows she will develop complications from having poor BG control. Vin hates being ill and people fussing over her, especially when they don't understand what's wrong and she can't make herself understood because her brain is confused with low glucose levels. Vin also feels that people don't understand why her personality is altered when she's hypo, so it's something she'd rather avoid; she keeps her BG around 12mml/L as she feels better mentally than if she's 5–6 mmol/L.

REDUCED PARTICIPATION IN SOCIAL EVENTS

Another issue for students away from home at college or university is the feeling that their diabetes has affected their ability to enjoy social events. This ties in with wanting to appear normal and avoid hypos in a social situation. Feeling able to join in has many issues attached to it such as having to restrict or avoid alcohol when there is pressure to drink and have a good time, having to watch BG levels if dancing is involved, not knowing the carbohydrate values of foods on offer at parties, and having to act and draw attention if hypos do happen, especially if friends feel they have to be responsible in this situation. Eating out and injecting at different times is also difficult, so many feel that it's easier to just enjoy themselves and not worry about diabetes. This strategy won't do any harm if it's only once in a while, but if it happens several times a week, this is not good diabetes self-management.

- Many students (if they are being honest) feel that they don't have good control of their diabetes at college or university.
- Students with diabetes often have problems balancing their health care and their educational needs.
- Rather than have a hypo in a classroom or social situation, many students with diabetes would rather run a higher BG to

avoid this risk, protecting them from this inconvenient situation.

- Many students with diabetes feel they receive little support from either their college/university or diabetes team, and they may have problems even getting an appointment during the holidays when they are not away from home studying.
- Individuals with diabetes may not wish to tell their peers about their condition because it's a hidden disability and they don't want to appear different.
- Students with diabetes may not join in with social events for fear of embarrassment over hypos, or they may 'ignore' their diabetes so they can have a good time with friends.

It is difficult to overcome these problems, especially if your child doesn't talk to you or the college/university about them. Paediatric diabetes teams could liaise with adult clinics to make the changeover easier for young adults, and this may help to identify difficulties such as arranging appointments when your young adult is at home. In this way your young adult will be able to discuss any problems they have had during their time away from home.

Issues for older people with diabetes

In the UK it is thought that by 2025, the number of people in their 80s and 90s will have doubled according to the World Health Organisation. Older people with diabetes have additional problems to the general older population such as having 70% higher rates of hospital admission. It's important to remember that older people might have had Type 1 diabetes all their life, they may have developed Type 2 diabetes in their 40s or 50s, or they may even be newly diagnosed. Because rates of Type 2 are so high at the moment, a distinction between Type 1 and Type 2 is no longer made and 'diabetes' has become a general term for everyone with the condition. Health professionals can also assume (they have done with me) that your diabetes is Type 2 because you are attending a diabetes clinic full of people with Type 2, rather than understanding that you've had Type 1 since childhood.

FACT: The Department of Health has stated that older people should be treated as individuals and enabled to make choices about their diabetes care.

If an older person has not lived their life with Type 1 diabetes (or developed Type 2 in their 40s or 50s) they may develop 'elderly onset' Type 2. Here, insulin is produced at a normal rate but it doesn't work as well, increasing BG levels. Type 2 diabetes is very common in older people because insulin is less effective, even when there is no obesity and the person is active. Because of this, BG levels become much higher than normal after meals.

Older people may not complain of the symptoms of Type 2 diabetes, or symptoms may not be noticed as they happen over many years. Particular symptoms of Type 2 in older people may be:

- Loss of appetite.
- Weakness.
- Weight loss.
- Loss of bladder control (usually due to the prostate gland pressing on the bladder in men and bladder and kidney infections in women).

FACT: Older people with untreated Type 2 diabetes may not have thirst as a symptom as their ability to feel thirst is altered.

While many older people with diabetes manage their condition very well, certain problems connected with old age can affect their control of BG:

MENTAL FUNCTIONING

Mental function in older persons may be impaired causing problems when. managing diabetes as it requires a high level of mental awareness: following a specific diet and medication regime, and some people have to test their blood glucose regularly. (This may not be the case if diabetes is diagnosed in an elderly person as the emphasis is not on keeping BG under control because complications are unlikely to develop within that person's lifetime). Studies have shown that there is a link between the development of dementia (loss of mental functioning) and having either Type 1 or Type 2 diabetes, making it much harder to carry out diabetes self-care tasks. If dementia or Alzheimer's disease is diagnosed, tests to determine mental functioning can show whether the person is able to live alone, or whether they need a carer to visit, sheltered housing or nursing home care.

DIET

Many older people with diabetes are able to care for themselves and may only have problems associated with getting proper nutrition. Preparing healthy meals can also be difficult because the older person has:

- A low income.

- Poor vision.
- Poor appetite due to decreased taste and smell.
- Arthritis or tremor (shaking) making food preparation difficult.
- Poor teeth or a dry mouth.
- Depression so that appetite is affected.
- Feels that they are too old to worry about caring for diabetes.

One or many of these problems may mean that the elderly person has an inadequate diet and poor diabetes control. Social Services (in the UK) can make sure one nutritious cooked meal suited to the diabetes diet is delivered to the individual's home every day. Some areas also provide meal choices for different ethnic backgrounds, and private companies provide meals by daily or weekly deliveries.

EXERCISE

If they have previously had a fit and healthy life, older people with diabetes may be concerned about diet and exercise. Exercise as a way of reducing BG may be limited, although exercise does lower BG and HbA1c in every age group. Because older people are more likely to have coronary heart disease, arthritis, eye disease, neuropathy (nerve damage) and reduced blood flow in the feet and legs any exercise must be gentle and not make any of these conditions worse. Help The Aged run local groups that allow the individual to participate in gentle exercise, and also to socialise with other people.

FACT: Older people with diabetes shouldn't end up in hospital unnecessarily because care home staff don't know how to look after them.

EYESIGHT

Eye disease is more likely to occur in older people who have diabetes, and this can make every aspect of their diabetes care more difficult. *Cataracts, macular degeneration*, and *glaucoma* are far more likely to develop, as well as diabetic retinopathy. Despite this, one-third of older people have never had their eyes examined, meaning these eye conditions are not diagnosed and treated early on. This is a serious problem and, according to Diabetes UK, the vast majority of cases of diabetes-related blindness can be prevented with early treatment.

URINARY AND SEXUAL PROBLEMS

Older people with diabetes are often affected by urinary and sexual problems. The bladder muscles can become paralysed so that urine can't be passed and, when the bladder becomes too full, the urine flows out. Mobility problems may also make it difficult to get to the toilet on time, and spasms in the bladder muscle may push urine out of the body. These problems can also cause frequent infections of the urinary tract.

Over 60% of men over 70 who have diabetes also have erectile dysfunction and 50% have no desire to have sex. It's thought that older men are likely to have blocked blood vessels, affecting blood flow to the penis. Various medications taken by older men may also affect sexual function, so if this is a problem it should be reported to the GP so that the cause can be investigated and treated

FACT: A study of 113 older people with Type 2 diabetes showed that 90% felt their BG-lowering medication was effective and necessary, but 60% were also worried about the long-term effects of their tablets and 25% felt some diabetes medications were over-prescribed by doctors.

MEDICATION

If diet and exercise can't be used to control an older person's BG, glucose-lowering medication will be considered. While this solves one problem it may present others, such as:

- Taking the wrong dosage of tablets because of poor eyesight.
- Lack of understanding about what the tablets are for and why they are important.
- Difficulty with getting the child-proof bottle open to take the tablets.
- Problems with different medications that are taken reacting with one another.
- The presence of liver or kidney impairment meaning the medication effects last longer.
- Poor appetite meaning the individual has frequent low BG.

When an older person prescribed BG-lowering tablets goes from looking after themselves to going into a care home, their dosages may need altering if they have not been taking the medication when they have been told to or in the right amounts.

FACT: It is important to remember that many older people are capable of administering their own medications and that they may be very independent in this respect.

Caring for people with diabetes

Current thinking (and I'm sure my husband would agree) suggests that living with and caring for someone with diabetes can be mentally challenging. When the person with diabetes has to provide information about their condition to health professionals, this greatly increases their partner's understanding of how that person copes with their diabetes and this, in turn, helps the partner/carer cope better. This involvement by another person also helps the individual with diabetes to manage their condition and carry out the self-care tasks they have to do. This knowledge of a partner's health problems is known as 'condition specific', meaning that they are confident and able to take part in the management of diabetes, improving the wellbeing of the whole family.

FACT: Knowledge and support from partners can improve diabetes self-management.

When a child or a young adult develops diabetes it becomes a family condition, where carbohydrates are counted at mealtimes, injections are taken at certain times and everyone knows the importance of this event, and family members are aware of what to do when the person with diabetes has a hypo or if they feel unwell. When a person with diabetes gets married, their partner learns about the condition and acts in the same way that the family does, supporting the person with diabetes when they need it. If the person with diabetes prefers to be independent, they may exclude their loved ones, or they may need more help with day-to-day tasks as they get older, putting demands on the relationship with their partner:

Case Study

Kathy Goldstein has been married to her husband, Joe, for 22 years. He had Type 1 diabetes when they met, so Kathy feels she has never known any different. Joe developed sight difficulties ten years ago and relies on Kathy when they go shopping to read labels and to do the driving. Katy feels that their relationship has changed from one where she relied on Joe to earn a wage and pay the bills to Kathy being a carer who has now taken over responsibility for a lot of the household chores. She doesn't mind this, but can see how some marriages might be affected by the progression of any chronic disease so that things become different. Kathy feels it's important for Joe to know he has her support, and for her to add alternative suggestions to certain life situations and diabetes-related problems that Joe hasn't thought of.

FACT: Whether or not a partner is prepared to become a carer depends on your relationship.

Case Study

Chris Marshall didn't give his partner, Lynn's, diabetes another thought when they were younger because she could drive, work, and look after herself and the house. When Lynn became pregnant in her late-twenties, Chris was concerned that her Type 1 diabetes would affect the baby, but because they were both still young, he didn't worry too much. Lynn had severe problems with her BG control during her pregnancy and she became more and more dependent on Chris to help around the house. Unfortunately, Lynn then had a miscarriage and she and Chris drifted apart when she really needed his support. Eventually they split up because Chris blamed Lynn for losing the baby due to her diabetes.

Some partners feel that diabetes represents a third person in the relationship, sometimes excluding them as the diabetes grabs the attention. This is especially the case when the person with diabetes speaks to others with the condition, discussing shared experiences and being members of 'the diabetes club'. Although people with diabetes like to talk to others who have been through similar experiences (as I have said before), how your partner reacts obviously depends on their personality and your relationship with them. Although diabetes is something that you have to deal with yourself, support from others with and without the condition is really necessary to help you cope and manage as well as possible. This might seem obvious, but some partners find the shared diabetes thing so frustrating that it causes conflict:

Case Study

Rav Nadim would get very irritated when his wife, Pria, invited her friends and family around to have a 'Type 2 diabetes party', where Pria would make carbohydrate-counted snacks and buy sugar-free drinks. Pria had four aunties with Type 2 and two friends that she'd met at diabetes clinic who would come along, and she enjoyed chatting about diabetes with them and exchanging recipes and information. Although Pria carried on arranging these get-togethers every couple of months, she wished Rav would join in and support her in having to live with Type 2. Pria made special meals for herself while the rest of the family ate as much as they liked, which upset her. It was difficult to come to a compromise because Rav wanted Pria to eat what she'd cooked for the family, and Pria wanted Rav to understand her condition – that she had to watch what she ate as she controlled her diabetes through diet, exercise and medication. In the end Pria's diabetes nurse was able to speak to Rav and explain the condition and the importance of diet to control BG. Rav was more supportive after that, explaining that he hadn't been *asked* to be involved in any of Pria's diabetes care or management.

Like all long-term (chronic) health conditions, diabetes affects the relationship between couples and families. It's thought that the emotional costs of living with someone with diabetes are high, especially with Type 1 because of the mood swings associated with low BG. This is because of the unpredictable nature of BG control, as well as feelings of irritation and frustration and the restrictions diabetes can pose to the lifestyle of the couple. Partners may experience isolation because of their partner's diabetes and if they also have a lack of knowledge about the condition, this will mean that the person with diabetes will be affected. This means that health professionals should understand that:

- The person with diabetes is not the only person who has to deal with it.
- Both the person with diabetes *and* their partner need to talk to other people who are going through the same problems.
- Involving both people in a relationship in diabetes discussions is reassuring for both.
- Education and support for partners/carers is needed to help deal with the diagnosis of diabetes in a loved one.

FACT: Partners have to feel they have some control over the condition too so that if the person can't do their insulin or a blood test, the carer knows what to do.

HELPFUL HINTS, RECIPES AND TIPS

'You definitely need to know where you can get some help to deal with it all'

There are things you can do to allow other people in so you can share your diabetes self-care with them – it helps them to feel valued, useful, and part of things and it helps you manage your condition.

- YOU must be responsible for managing your diabetes on a day-to-day basis.
- You should participate in agreeing your self-care goals and treatment plan with your diabetes team and take the advice you're given seriously.
- Tell your employer you have diabetes and make sure the people you work with know how to treat a hypo.
- Teach your friends and relatives how to recognise a hypo (make a list of symptoms and pass it round!) and what they should do if you have one.
- Keep your BG as near-normal as you can (between 5–7 mmol/L) to avoid the onset of complications. Make sure you have an annual eye examination, blood, urine and nerve tests, and regular foot checks. It is YOUR responsibility to make sure these are done.
- Exercise regularly with a friend or relatives – walk the dog together or go swimming with someone. Having a commitment to meet up will help you do planned exercise and not put it off.
- Make sure you have the contact details for a DIRECT ACCESS chiropodist if you suddenly develop a problem with

your feet and you need to refer yourself to someone who can help as soon as possible. You can get these details from your GP surgery.

- Tell your family what you should be eating so they can help prepare the right foods and you can find restaurants together that serve healthy options rather than high-fat, high-calorie meals. If other people are also eating healthy options, you don't feel like you're missing out.

- Once you've come to terms with your diagnosis and have accepted that you have diabetes, you should receive a course of diabetes education as this is vital for you to manage your condition properly. If you haven't received this already, ask your diabetes team or your GP for information.

- Make sure you know how your diabetes medication works, how long it works for, and when it might not work properly (such as if it's taken with other medications).

- Work with a dietician so you can still enjoy your favourite foods. The dietician in your diabetes team wants to help make having diabetes as easy as possible for you so it fits into your lifestyle as painlessly as possible.

- Make sure you are up to date with advances in diabetes care as things are changing all the time and new developments become reality. You can discuss this with your diabetes team and/or GP. Remember – if you don't ask, you don't get!

Recipes

Some self-help books about diabetes contain recipes using swordfish, morel, chanterelle, and couscous (I'm not saying which ones, but this doesn't seem like the type of meal the average person would cook on a day-to-day basis). When a person is diagnosed with diabetes, and once they've been taught what they should and shouldn't be eating, it can be difficult to think of meal solutions that won't drastically increase BG levels.

If you really want to get into diabetes-friendly cooking in a serious way there are many excellent cookbooks available that cover this subject. TIP: Have a flick through before you buy to see if you actually fancy eating some of the suggested meals, as well as finding out if they are easy and quick to make and suit your pocket. I have shared some of my favourite recipe suggestions from the Diabetes UK website for breakfast, lunch, dinner and treats below, including the carbohydrate and calorie content of each meal, the sugar, fat and salt content, and how much of the daily five recommended portions of fruit or veg each contains.

FACT: It's important that you enjoy your food!

Breakfast solutions
APRICOT PORRIDGE WITH TOASTED SEEDS

Serves 2

Preparation time: 15 minutes

Cooking time: 10 minutes

Half of the porridge contains: 34.6 grams of carbohydrate; 219 calories; 17.0 grams of sugars; 5.8 grams of fat; less than 0.1 grams of salt; and half a portion of fruit.

Ingredients:

50 grams of ready-to-eat dried apricots

150 millilitres of orange or apple juice

50 grams of porridge oats

15 grams of mixed seeds such as pumpkin, sesame and poppy seeds

Method:

1. Place the apricots in a small saucepan and cover with the fruit juice. Bring to the boil and simmer for 5 minutes.

2. Set the apricots aside for 10 minutes, then place them in a food processor or blender and blend to a purée.

3. Place the oats in a small saucepan and cover with 600 millilitres of water and place over a low heat to cook for 3–4 minutes. Toast a quarter of a cup of mixed seeds under the grill.

4. Stir half the apricot purée into the porridge and divide between two bowls. Top with the toasted seeds and a swirl of purée.

POTATO PANCAKES

Makes 12

Preparation time: 25 minutes

Cooking time: 25 minutes

Each 54 gram serving contains 9.6 grams of carbohydrate; 67 calories; less than 0.5 grams of sugars; 1.8 grams of fat; and 0.2 grams of salt.

Ingredients:

450 grams of potatoes, peeled and chopped

3 eggs, yolks beaten, whites separated

Freshly grated nutmeg to taste

50 grams of self-raising flour

2 egg whites

Salt and freshly ground black pepper

A little sunflower/oil for frying

Method:

1. Boil the potatoes for 10–12 minutes, or until tender. Drain and mash well (or press through a potato ricer). Leave to cool completely, then stir in the beaten egg yolks and nutmeg and season well.

2. Whisk the egg whites until they form soft peaks, then gently fold into the potato mixture. Heat a little oil in a non-stick frying pan, form the mixture into 12 pancakes and cook until golden brown.

3. Place on a piece of kitchen paper to absorb any excess oil, then serve.

TASTY TOASTIES

Serves 4

Preparation time: 10 minutes

Cooking time: 10 minutes

Each 184 gram serving contains 35.3 grams of carbohydrate; 294 calories; 3.3 grams of sugars; 11 grams of fat; 1.6 grams of salt; and 1 portion of vegetables.

Ingredients:

1 wholemeal baguette cut into 16 slices (1.5 centimetres thick)

8 cherry tomatoes, sliced

1 red pepper, thinly sliced

4 mushrooms, sliced

1 slice of lean ham cut into strips

70 grams of cooked spinach, water squeezed out

2 spring onions, finely sliced

2 eggs, scrambled

75 grams reduced-fat mature Cheddar cheese, finely grated

Method:

1. Prepare all your ingredients and assemble a selection of toppings.

2. Lay baguette slices on a grill pan and toast one side, remove and turn the bread over.

3. Arrange the toppings on the baguette slices and make a few of each.

4. Sprinkle each slice with a little grated Cheddar.

5. Grill until starting to brown, then serve.

MINI BLUEBERRY PANCAKES

Makes 10 pancakes

Preparation time: 10 minutes

Cooking time: 15–20 minutes

Each 74 gram serving contains 16.3 grams of carbohydrate; 100 calories; 2.8 grams of sugars; 1.8 grams of fat; 0.2 grams of salt; and ½ a portion of fruit.

Ingredients:

200 grams of wholemeal flour

1 teaspoon of baking powder

1 medium egg, beaten

250 millilitres of skimmed milk

1 teaspoon of vanilla extract

200 grams of fresh blueberries

2 teaspoons of sunflower oil

1 teaspoon of sugar substitute

Method:

1. Mix the flour and baking powder in a bowl.

2. In a separate bowl, beat together the egg, milk and vanilla extract.

3. Make a well in the middle of the flour, then gradually stir in the egg and milk mixture until you get a smooth batter.

4. Ideally, leave to stand for a few minutes before cooking.

5. Lightly crush half the blueberries with a fork and mix these into the batter along with the remaining (whole) blueberries.

6. Add a little oil to a non-stick frying-pan, then add the batter to the pan making sure the blueberries are evenly distributed.

7. Cook the pancakes on a medium heat for 2–3 minutes then turn them and cook for a further 2 minutes. *The pancakes are ready to turn when you see bubbles appearing on the surface. Sprinkle with a little sugar substitute before serving with some low-fat yoghurt or crème fraiche if liked.

MICROWAVE IN A MUG: APPLE AND CINNAMON FRUITY PORRIDGE

Serves 1

Preparation time: 2 minutes

Cooking time: 2 minutes

Each 244 serving contains 34 grams of carbohydrate; 202 calories; 37 grams of fat; 10.2 grams of sugars; 0.01 grams of salt; and 1 portion of fruit.

Ingredients:

35 grams of porridge oats

1 teaspoon of cinnamon (and a pinch for the top)

1 teaspoon of artificial sweetener

1 small apple, chopped small

25 millilitres of semi-skimmed milk

Method:

1. Add oats, sweetener, cinnamon and apple to a mug.

2. Add 100 millilitres of water and cook on full power (800 watts) for 2 minutes.

3. Add the milk, mix and sprinkle over a little cinnamon.

Lovely lunches

MUSHROOM AND SPRING ONION OMELETTE

Serves 1

Preparation time: 5 minutes

Cooking time: 10 minutes

The omelette contains 3 grams of carbohydrate; 251 calories; 2.5 grams of sugars; 16.5 grams of fat; 0.7 grams of salt; and 2 portions of vegetables.

Ingredients:

2 eggs

Pinch of white pepper

1 teaspoon of sunflower oil

150 grams of mushrooms, sliced

1 spring onion, chopped

10 grams of reduced-fat Cheddar cheese

Method:

1. Break the eggs into a bowl, add pepper and beat with a fork. Set aside.

2. Heat the oil in a frying pan and cook the mushrooms and spring onion for 5 minutes on a medium-heat, stirring regularly until soft.

3. Stir the eggs into the mushrooms and spring onion for one minute, then cook gently for 3 minutes. Use a spatula to ease the omelette from the sides of the frying pan.

4. When the omelette is cooked, sprinkle the cheese on top and turn it out onto a plate, folding it in half.

CAULIFLOWER PIZZA (GLUTEN FREE)

Serves 2

Preparation time: 30 minutes

Cooking time: 30 minutes

Half of the pizza contains 18 grams of carbohydrate; 382 calories; 34.8 grams of sugars; 18.1 grams of fat; 0.5 grams of salt; and 3 portions of vegetables

Ingredients:

1 cauliflower

2 teaspoons of sunflower oil

75 grams of red onion, thinly sliced

150 grams of courgette, diced

2 fresh tomatoes, chopped

2 cloves of garlic, crushed

1 heaped teaspoon of dried oregano

1 egg, beaten

25 grams of Parmesan cheese, finely grated

80 grams of reduced-fat Mozzarella cheese, thinly sliced

6–8 fresh bay leaves, torn

½ teaspoon of chilli flakes (optional)

Method:

1. Pre-heat oven to 180 degrees centigrade, Gas mark 4. Remove stalks from the cauliflower and break into pieces. Hand grate or blitz in a food processor.

2. Add cauliflower to a bowl and cover with cling-film, piercing the film a few times. Cook in a microwave on high for 4–5 minutes (or steam cauliflower for 2 minutes). Allow to cool.

3. Once cauliflower is completely cool, place it onto a clean tea towel and press over the sink to remove any excess water.

4. Make pizza topping: heat the oil in a frying pan and cook the onion, red pepper and courgette for 4–5 minutes until starting to brown. Add tomatoes, garlic and oregano and cook for another 2 minutes. Mix well and set aside.

5. Add cauliflower to a bowl with the egg and Parmesan and mix well.

6. Line a round baking tray or pizza sheet (25 centimetres in diameter) with non-stick baking paper and spread the cauliflower mixture to the thickness of ¾ of a centimetre onto it. Bake for 15 minutes. Add topping and serve sprinkled with bay leaves and chilli flakes (if using).

FRENCH ONION SOUP

Serves 4

Preparation time: 15 minutes

Cooking time: 45 minutes

Each 590 gram serving contains 54.8 grams of carbohydrate; 287 calories; 23 grams of sugars; 5.8 grams of fat; 0.9 grams of salt; and 4 portions of vegetables.

Ingredients:

3 teaspoons of sunflower oil

1 kilogram of onions, finely chopped

400 grams of sweet potato, cut into wedges

1 low-salt vegetable stock cube dissolved in 800 millilitres of boiling water

4 slices of wholemeal bread (30 grams per slice)

20 grams of reduced-fat mature Cheddar cheese

20 grams of Mozzarella cheese

1 tablespoon of fresh parsley, finely chopped, plus extra to serve

1 teaspoon of low-salt soy sauce

Good pinch of white pepper

Method:

1. Pre-heat the oven to 190 degrees centigrade or Gas mark 5. Add 2 teaspoons of oil to a saucepan then add the onions and cook over a very low heat for 30–40 minutes, stirring regularly so the onions caramelise.

2. While the onions are caramelising, pour the remaining oil onto a baking sheet. Add the potatoes and move them around until they're coated in oil. Bake in oven for 30–40 minutes.

3. Add the stock to the onions, bring to the boil and simmer for 5 minutes.

4. For the cheesy croutons: cut each slice of bread in half and grill, then turn over and top each piece with Cheddar cheese and Mozzarella and grill again until cheese melts and browns. Alternatively, you can put the cheese-topped bread on a baking tray and cook in the oven for 5–10 minutes.

5. Stir in the parsley, pepper and soy sauce, then place in four bowls. Serve with cheesy croutons and a sprinkling of fresh parsley on top, with the potato wedges on the side.

CAESAR SALAD WITH CHAR-GRILLED CHICKEN

Serves 4
Preparation time: 10 minutes
Cooking time: 16 minutes
Each 229 gram serving contains 37.1 grams of carbohydrate; 350 calories; 4.8 grams of sugars; 11.5 grams of fat; and 1.4 grams of salt.

Ingredients:
For the dressing:

30 grams of Parmesan cheese, finely grated

2 teaspoons of low-fat yoghurt

1 tablespoon of extra virgin olive oil

1 tablespoon Dijon mustard

Juice of ¼ of a lemon

1 teaspoon of Worcestershire sauce

Pinch of white pepper

For the salad:

80 grams of little gem lettuce

2 skinless and boneless chicken breasts

1 teaspoon of olive oil

For the croutons:

1 clove of garlic, crushed

½ a tablespoon of olive oil

Pinch of black pepper

10 centimetre length of baguette or ciabatta bread, cubed

10 grams of Parmesan cheese shavings to top

Method:

1. Pre-heat the oven to 180 degrees centigrade or Gas mark 4. Mix all of the dressing ingredients together and leave to infuse.

2. For the salad, break the lettuce into individual leaves, wash and thoroughly drain.

3. Slice the chicken breasts in half to make them thinner. Rub with a little oil, then cook on a hot griddle pan for 2–3 minutes each side, or until thoroughly cooked through, then cut into strips.

4. To make the croutons, add the garlic and olive oil to a bowl and crush further with the back of a spoon. Add the black pepper, mix well and coat the insides of the bowl with the mixture.

5. Add the bread cubes and mix so all the bread is coated with some of the oil. Spread the cubes onto a baking tray and bake in the pre-heated oven for around 8–10 minutes, turning a couple of times with a spatula and being careful not to burn them.

6. To assemble, layer the lettuce in a shallow bowl, saving the smaller leaves until last so you create concentric circles. Drizzle with the dressing, sprinkle with the croutons and chicken, and top with Parmesan shavings.

CREAMY BACON AND ROSEMARY PASTA

Serves 2

Preparation time: 10 minutes

Cooking time: 10–12 minutes

Each 38 gram serving contains 71.6 grams of carbohydrate; 472 calories; 8.3 grams of sugars; 10.4 grams of fat; 1.8 grams of salt; and one portion of vegetables.

Ingredients:

175 grams of dried pasta shapes

2 rashers of lean back bacon, chopped

1 leek (150 grams), finely chopped

1 teaspoon of fresh rosemary, chopped

1 carton of natural yoghurt

1 tablespoon of sundried tomato paste

Freshly ground black pepper to taste

A little fresh grated Parmesan to top the finished pasta

Method:

1. Cook the pasta according to the pack instructions, then drain.

2. Meanwhile, place the bacon into a frying pan and fry for 2 minutes (adding no extra oil); then add the leeks and rosemary and fry for a further 3–4 minutes until the leek is cooked.

3. Mix the yoghurt and sundried tomato paste and stir into the pasta, adding the bacon and the rosemary. Sprinkle a little Parmesan cheese on the top and serve with plenty of salad vegetables.

Mouth-watering main meals

BEEF GOULASH

Serves 2

Preparation time: 15 minutes

Cooking time: 2 hours

Half of the goulash contains 36.6 grams of carbohydrate; 370 calories; 12.7 grams of sugars; 8.7 grams of fat; 1.7 grams of salt; and 2.3 portions of vegetables.

Ingredients:

250 grams of lean braising steak

250 grams of new potatoes

2 teaspoons of seasoned flour (with black pepper and small amount of salt substitute added to taste)

1 teaspoon of sunflower oil

1 onion, chopped

½ red pepper, chopped

1 clove garlic, crushed

1 teaspoon paprika

200 grams can of chopped tomatoes

1 teaspoon of tomato purée

150 millilitres (¼ of a pint) of beef stock

Method:

1. Preheat the oven to 180 degrees centigrade or Gas mark 4.

2. Toss the steak in the seasoned flour. Heat the oil in a flame-proof casserole dish, add the steak and fry for 2–3 minutes until brown all over.

3. Add the remaining ingredients and bring to the boil, then put the lid on the casserole dish and place in the oven for 1½ – 2 hours until the meat is tender.

4. Serve with plenty of vegetables.

SPINACH AND RICOTTA CANNELONI

Serves 6

Preparation time: 30 minutes

Cooking time: 25 minutes

Each 170 gram serving contains: 20 grams of carbohydrate; 160 calories; 4.8 grams of fat; 5.5 grams of sugar; 0.3 grams of salt; and 1 portion of vegetables.

Ingredients:

1 teaspoon of sunflower oil

1 large onion, finely chopped

1 leek, finely chopped

3 cloves of garlic, crushed

250 grams of frozen leaf spinach

150 grams of ricotta cheese

½ teaspoon nutmeg

120 grams of cannelloni pasta (dry weight) cooked according to pack instructions. After cooking, keep the pasta moist with some cold water

400 gram tin of chopped tomatoes

1 tablespoon oregano

1 tablespoon of tomato purée

A generous grind of black pepper

25 grams of Mozzarella cheese, thinly sliced

Method:

1. Pre-heat oven to 180 degrees centigrade or Gas mark 4. Add the oil to a saucepan and cook the onion and leek for 5–8

minutes. Mix in the garlic and cook together for another couple of minutes before removing from the heat.

2. Add the spinach, ricotta cheese and nutmeg and mix well.

3. Put the tinned tomatoes in a bowl and add the oregano, tomato purée and black pepper. Mix together to make the sauce.

4. Stuff the spinach and ricotta mixture into the cannelloni. Put half the tomato sauce in an ovenproof dish. Place the stuffed cannelloni on top and add the remaining sauce. Top with Mozzarella and bake for 15 minutes.

ZINGY SALMON FILLETS

Serves 6

Preparation time: 10 minutes

Cooking time: 8 minutes

Each 141 gram serving of salmon contains 2.7 grams of carbohydrate; 246 calories; 25 grams of sugars; 15 grams of fat; and 1.1 grams of salt.

Ingredients:

6 pieces of skinless salmon fillet (approximately 125 grams each)

For the marinade:

2 tablespoons of soy sauce

2 teaspoons of sesame oil

A pinch of chilli flakes

1 teaspoon of ginger, grated

Garnish:

1 tablespoon of freshly chopped coriander

4 spring onions, sliced

Method:

1. Place the marinade ingredients into a non-metallic bowl and stir well.

2. Add the salmon fillets and coat in the marinade. Set aside for the flavours to infuse.

3. Cook for 3–4 minutes on a medium heat then add any remaining marinade, turning the salmon over to cook the other side for 3–4 minutes. Scatter over the coriander and spring onions before serving.

BUBBLE AND SQUEAK (GLUTEN FREE)

Serves 3

Preparation time: 15 minutes

Cooking time: 30 minutes

Each 336-gram portion contains 31.2 grams of carbohydrate; 325 calories; 8.7 grams of sugars; 15.9 grams of fat; 0.6 grams of salt; and 1.5 portions of vegetables.

Ingredients:

350 grams of potatoes, cubed

1 large parsnip, peeled and cubed

4 tablespoons of milk

25 grams of low-fat spread

1 teaspoon of sunflower oil

1 small onion, chopped

1 large carrot, peeled and grated

100 grams of green cabbage, finely shredded

3 medium eggs

Salt substitute and freshly ground black pepper

Method:

1. Cook the potatoes and parsnips together in boiling water for 12–15 minutes, or until tender. Drain and mash with the milk and low-fat spread. Season well.

2. Heat the oil in a medium frying pan. Add the onion, carrot and cabbage and fry for 5 minutes.

3. Add the vegetables to the mashed potatoes and form 3 patties. Fry for 4–5 minutes, turning the patties halfway through the cooking.

4. Poach the eggs and serve on top of the bubble and squeak.

FISH PIE

Serves 6

Preparation time: 6 minutes

Cooking time: 45–55 minutes

Each 382 gram serving contains 36.9 grams of carbohydrate; 339 calories; 12.8 grams of sugars; 8.4 grams of fat; 0.9 grams of salt; and 2 portions of vegetables.

Ingredients:

1 kilogram of sweet potatoes

2 teaspoons of sunflower oil

2 leeks, halved lengthways, then chopped

1 heaped teaspoon of plain flour

1 fish stock cube

400 millilitres of skimmed milk

Good pinch of white pepper

25 grams of fresh parsley (save some for garnishing)

1 heaped teaspoon paprika

300 grams of Pollack fish, cut into cubes

300 grams of salmon, cut into cubes

Pinch of black pepper

Method:

1. Pre-heat the oven to 180 degrees centigrade or Gas mark 4. Boil the sweet potatoes for 15–20 minutes until soft, then drain.

2. Heat the oil in a saucepan over a low to medium heat and fry the leeks, stirring regularly until soft (7 minutes).

3. Sprinkle the flour over the leeks and crumble the stock cube over. Mix well for a minute or so until the leeks are coated.

4. Slowly stir in ¼ of the milk until it becomes quite thick, then gradually add in the rest stirring constantly until it comes to the boil. Stir in the white pepper and parsley and remove from heat.

5. Mash the sweet potatoes thoroughly and mix with the paprika.

6. Add the leek sauce to an oven-proof dish and arrange the fish so that it's evenly distributed. Top with the sweet potato and bake for 25–35 minutes until the sauce starts to bubble through the sweet potato. Sprinkle with parsley and black pepper.

Delightful desserts

APPLE CHARLOTTE

Serves 4

Preparation time: 10 minutes

Cooking time: 20 minutes

Each 180 gram serving contains: 27.6 grams of carbohydrate; 162 calories; 7.4 grams of sugar; 3.2 grams of fat; 0.5 grams of salt; and 1 portion of fruit.

Ingredients:

3 unpeeled apples, cored and grated.

200 millilitres of apple juice

1 tablespoon of Blackstrap molasses sugar (molasses are processed to remove most of the sugar)

2 teaspoons cinnamon

A dash of sunflower oil

4–5 slices of wholemeal bread with crusts removed

1 egg yolk, lightly beaten

Method:

1. Pre-heat oven to 180 degrees centigrade or Gas mark 4. Add the apples to a saucepan with half (100 millilitres) of the apple juice and simmer until soft (4-5 minutes). Leaving the juice in the pan, place the apples in a bowl.

2. Add the molasses sugar and cinnamon to the pan with the remaining 100 millilitres of apple juice and gently melt the sugar, adding a little more juice if needed. Allow to cool (this should make around 100 millilitres of syrup.

3. Rub the sunflower oil around a small pudding basin and line the basin with the bread (keeping some for the top of the Charlotte). Pour the syrup into the basin, keeping some to pour over to soak the bread on the top.

4. Stir the egg yolk and the apple together and put the mixture into the pudding basin. Top with the remaining bread and pour on the last of the syrup. Spoon over any remaining liquid.

5. Bake for 20 minutes (check after 15 minutes and if the top of the Charlotte is very brown at the edges, place a piece of foil over the top for the remaining 5 minutes).

6. Allow to stand for a couple of minutes before loosening the Charlotte with a knife around the edge of the basin. Carefully turn the Charlotte out onto a serving plate. You could serve this with a little low-fat plain yoghurt or low-fat crème fraiche.

BLACKCURRANT AND RASPBERRY ICE CREAM

Serves 4

Preparation time: 15 minutes, plus 2½ hours for freezing.

Cooking time: 15 minutes

Each 313 gram serving contains 28.9 grams of carbohydrate; 312 calories; 31.4 grams of sugar; 8.1 grams of fat; 0.2 grams of salt; and one portion of fruit.

Ingredients:

600 millilitres of unsweetened soya milk

Few drops of vanilla extract

1 tablespoon of cornflour

4 egg yolks

2 tablespoons of confectioner's sugar (a sugar-free alternative to icing sugar)

300 gram can of blackcurrants (in own juice) drained

200 grams of frozen raspberries

Method:

1. Place the milk and vanilla extract into a medium-sized saucepan and bring to the boil.

2. In a bowl, whisk together the cornflour, egg yolks and icing sugar.

3. Pour the milk over the cornflour mixture and stir in. Place over a low heat and cook until the mixture thickens. DO NOT boil, otherwise the mixture will curdle.

4. Cool the mixture, then stir in the blackcurrants and raspberries.

5. Transfer to a freezer-proof container.

6. Freeze for 2 hours, then beat with a fork to remove ice crystals. Return to freezer for 5–10 minutes before serving.

COCONUT RICE PUDDING

Serves 3–4

Preparation time: 10 minutes

Cooking time: 25 minutes

Each 210 gram serving contains 32 grams of carbohydrate; 179 calories; 6 grams of sugars; 4 grams of fat; 0.3 grams of salt; and no portions of fruit or vegetables.

Ingredients:

100 grams of Basmati rice

1 x 400 millilitre can of reduced-fat coconut milk

300 millilitres of soya milk

25 grams of granulated sugar substitute

Few drops of vanilla extract

1 tablespoon of toasted coconut

Method:

1. Place all the ingredients (except the toasted coconut) into a small saucepan. Place over a low heat and simmer very gently for 20–30 minutes until the rice is tender.

2. Top with toasted coconut and s

BLUEBERRY AND LEMON CHEESECAKE

Serves 1

Preparation time: 5 minutes

Each cheesecake contains 33.9 grams of carbohydrate; 279 calories; 19 grams of sugars; 11.5 grams of fat; 1.1 grams of salt; and 1 portion of fruit.

Ingredients:

Zest of ½ a lemon, finely grated, plus 1 teaspoon of lemon juice

1 heaped teaspoon of lemon curd

1 heaped teaspoon of reduced-fat cream cheese (approximately 60 grams)

75 grams of blueberries

2 oat cakes, crushed

Method:

1. Mix the lemon zest, lemon curd and cream cheese together in a bowl.

2. Gently crush half the blueberries with a fork and add lemon juice.

3. Add the remaining blueberries to the cream cheese and lemon curd mixture.

4. Place the crushed blueberries at the bottom of a serving glass. Top with the lemon cheese and sprinkle with oat cake crumbs. Garnish with lemon zest and remaining blueberries.

BERRY TRIFLE

Serves 8–10

Preparation time: 25 minutes, plus 2 hours cooling time

Cooking time: 15 minutes

Each 164 gram serving of trifle contains 9 grams of carbohydrate; 120 calories; 4.1 grams of sugars; 6.8 grams of fat; 0.2 grams of salt; and 1 portion of fruit.

Ingredients:

For the sponge:

40 grams of wholemeal flour

½ a teaspoon of baking powder

5 teaspoons of granulated sweetener

2 tablespoons of light olive oil and 1 teaspoon to oil the dish

1 small egg, beaten

1 teaspoon of vanilla extract

For the custard:

250 millilitres of skimmed milk, plus 2 teaspoons of semi-skimmed milk

20 grams of cornflour

1 teaspoon of vanilla extract

5 teaspoons of granulated sweetener

For the jelly:

1 x 23-gram sachet of sugar-free strawberry jelly crystals

300 grams of frozen mixed berries (don't defrost)

For the topping:

200 grams of 0% fat Greek yoghurt

200 grams of half-fat crème fraiche

10 grams of toasted flaked almonds

Grated zest of one lemon

Method:

1. To make the sponge: in a bowl, mix together the flour, baking powder and sweetener. Add the 2 teaspoons of oil, the egg and the vanilla extract and mix thoroughly until smooth.

2. Add 50 millilitres of water and beat. Lightly oil a one-pint microwave-proof bowl and pour the mixture in.

3. Microwave on full power (800 watts) for 2 minutes, 20 seconds, then allow to cool.

4. To make the custard, add 250 millilitres of skimmed milk to a saucepan and bring to boiling point.

5. Add the cornflour, vanilla extract, sweetener and 2 teaspoons of milk to a cup and mix well until smooth.

6. Once the milk is about to boil, stir in the cornflour mixture, stirring continuously with a wooden spoon and bring to boiling

point, stirring until thickened. Remove from the heat and leave to cool.

7. To assemble, break the sponge into pieces and scatter on the bottom of a glass bowl.

8. Make the jelly according to the instructions on the pack but use 10% less water than stated. Set aside and allow to cool for 10 minutes.

9. Scatter the berries on top of the sponge (use from frozen as this helps the jelly to set quicker).

10. Pour the jelly over the fruit and sponge, then place in the fridge for 30 minutes.

11. Spread custard over the jelly and return trifle to the fridge for 30 minutes. Cover with cling-film and leave in fridge overnight if wished.

12. To finish the trifle, mix the yoghurt and the crème fraiche together and use to top the custard, then scatter with almonds and lemon zest.

Tasty treats
RICH FRUIT CAKE (* This also makes an excellent Christmas cake)
Serves 12

Preparation time: 20 minutes

Cooking time: 1 – 1½ hours

Each 97 gram serving contains 24.8 grams of carbohydrate; 197 calories; 4.3 grams of sugars; 8.4 grams of fat; 0.2 grams of salt; and 1 portion of fruit and vegetables.

Ingredients:

75 grams of sultanas

100 grams of raisings

250 grams of candied peel

100 millilitres of boiling water

1 banana (100 grams) mashed

2 eggs, beaten

75 millilitres of sunflower oil

1 courgette (200 grams) grated

1 apple (100 grams) grated

1 carrot (80 grams) finely grated

150 grams of wholemeal flour

1 teaspoon of baking powder

3 teaspoons of mixed spice

6 glace cherries

20 grams of whole blanched almonds

Method:

1. Pre-heat the oven to 170 degrees centigrade or Gas mark 3. Add sultanas, raisins and peel to a bowl. Cover with boiling water and set aside.

2. Mix together the mashed banana, eggs and oil in a large bowl and beat well.

3. Mix the courgette, apple and carrot, then stir in the flour, baking powder and mixed spice. Next, add the dried fruit plus the soaking water.

4. Mix well and put into a 20 centimetre cake tin lined with baking parchment. Top mixture with cherries and almonds, cover with foil and bake for 1 –1½ hours. Remove the foil 15–20 minutes before the end of cooking time, then bake for the remainder of the time to brown the top.

5. Test with a skewer or knife (which should come out clean when the cake is cooked) and then remove from the oven.

CHEESE, ONION AND SPINACH SCONES
Makes 10
Preparation time: 15 minutes
Cooking time: 15 minutes
Each 44 gram serving contains 14.7 grams of carbohydrate; 113 calories; 0.7 grams of sugars; 3.9 grams of fat; and 0.2 grams of salt.

Ingredients:
200 grams of wholemeal flour
1 teaspoon of baking powder
Good pinch of white pepper

50 grams of mature low-fat Cheddar, grated, reserving 2 teaspoons

4 spring onions, chopped finely

75 grams of frozen spinach, defrosted with excess water removed to leave 50 grams

½ a teaspoon of paprika, optional

Method:

1. Pre-heat the oven to 180 degrees centigrade, Gas mark 4, then place a large baking tray in the oven.

2. Mix the flour, baking powder and pepper together, add the spinach and spring onion, then sprinkle grated cheese into the mixture to distribute it evenly.

3. Make a well in the centre of the mixture and pour in the oil and half the milk. Mix together and add the remaining milk until you have a soft but firm dough.

4. Lightly flour the surface and gently roll the dough until 2 centimetres thick. Cut out the scones with a medium cutter and then place on the hot oven tray. Pull together any scraps of dough and roll out again to get an extra couple of scones.

5. Glaze the tops of the scones with the extra milk and sprinkle with a little cheese and paprika (if wished).

6. Bake for 12–15 minutes until golden brown.

BLACKBERRY AND APPLE CAKE

Makes 12 slices

Preparation time: 10 minutes

Cooking time: 35–40 minutes

Each 72 gram serving contains 17.7 grams of carbohydrate; 156 calories; 7.3 grams of sugars; 7.5 grams of fat; and 0.1 grams of salt.

Ingredients:

2 apples

2 medium eggs

1 teaspoon of vanilla extract

75 grams of granulated sweetener

100 millilitres of sunflower oil (use one teaspoon for greasing the loaf tin)

150 grams of wholemeal flour

1 teaspoon of baking powder

150 grams of blackberries

Method:

1. Pre-heat the oven to 180 degrees centigrade or Gas mark 4. Use one teaspoon of oil to grease the loaf tin.

2. Grate the unpeeled apples into a bowl and discard the cores.

3. Add the eggs, vanilla extract, sugar substitute and oil to the bowl and beat together.

4. Add the flour and baking powder and mix well. Fold in the blackberries.

5. Pour the mixture into a loaf tin and bake for 25 minutes until firm and golden. Cover with foil after 20 minutes if it's starting to brown too much. The cake is cooked when a knife inserted into the centre comes out clean.

CHERRY AND CHOCOLATE DELIGHT
Serves 4
Preparation time: 20 minutes
Cooking time: 20 minutes
Each 109 gram serving contains 19 grams of carbohydrate; 114 calories; 8 grams of sugars; 2.2 grams of fat; 0.1 grams of salt; and half a portion of fruit.

Ingredients:
225 grams of fresh cherries
2 tablespoons of artificial sweetener
1 level teaspoon of cornflour blended with 1 teaspoon of cold water
100 grams of quark or low-fat soft cheese
2 tablespoons of skimmed milk
½ teaspoon of vanilla extract

For the chocolate sauce:
25 grams of dark chocolate, broken into pieces
1 heaped teaspoon of unsweetened cocoa powder (not drinking chocolate)

½ teaspoon of cornflour, blended with ½ teaspoon of cold water

1 level teaspoon of Blackstrap molasses sugar

Method:

1. Halve the cherries and remove the stones, reserving 4 whole cherries for decoration.

2. Put the halved cherries into a pan with 50 millilitres of water. Add a teaspoon of artificial sweetener. Simmer for 34 minutes until soft.

3. Blend the cornflour and cold water together and stir into the cherries until thickened.

4. Remove from heat and cool, stirring to prevent a skin forming.

5. In a bowl, beat the low-fat soft cheese, skimmed milk, vanilla extract and remaining sweetener together until smooth.

6. For the chocolate sauce: put the dark chocolate pieces into a small saucepan and add the unsweetened cocoa powder, the cornflour blended with water, and the molasses sugar. Heat, stirring constantly, until smooth. Cool, stirring to prevent a skin forming.

7. Spoon everything into 4 small serving glasses. Finish with a cherry, chill and serve.

OATY GINGER BISCUITS

Makes 24

Preparation time: 10 minutes

Cooking time: 25 minutes

Each 22 gram serving contains 7.1 grams of carbohydrate; 56 calories; 1.3 grams of sugars; 2.0 grams of fat; and 0.1 grams of salt.

Ingredients:

50 millilitres of sunflower oil

10 grams of Blackstrap molasses sugar

100 millilitres of skimmed milk

100 grams of wholemeal flour

1 level teaspoon of baking powder

3 teaspoons of powdered ginger

1 teaspoon of mixed spice

8 teaspoons of artificial sweetener

1 egg, beaten

1 ripe banana, mashed

Method:

1. Pre-heat oven to 150 degrees centigrade or Gas mark 2. Place the oil, molasses and milk in a saucepan and heat gently for 2 minutes.

2. In a bowl, mix together the flour, oatmeal, baking powder, ginger, mixed spice, and sweetener. Beat the egg and mashed banana and add.

3. Line a 300 centimetre baking tray with baking parchment. Gently stir the oil into the mixture and pour into the lined tin until about one centimetre thick. Bake in the centre of the oven for one hour, or until the centre of the mixture is firm to the touch.

4. Remove from the oven and leave it to cool in the tin for 15–20 minutes. Transfer to a chopping board and cut into squares.

Useful contacts

DIABETES UK

Tel: 0207 4241000 (language line available)

Minicom: 0207 4622757

Website: www.diabetes.org.uk

Email: info@diabetes.org.uk

THE DIABETES FEDERATION OF IRELAND

Aims to help people with diabetes and their families

www.diabetesireland.ie

DIABETES IN SCOTLAND

Provides information about diabetes and it treatment.

www.diabetecotland.org

HEALTH OF WALES INFORMATION SERVICE (HOWIS)

Provides health and lifestyle information for the population of Wales.

www.wales.nhs.uk

THE AMERICAN DIABETES ASSOCIATION

Tel: 800-342-2383

Website: www.diabetes.org

DOSAGNE ADJUSTMENT FOR NORMAL EATING (DAFNE)

http://www.dafne.uk.com

ROYAL NATIONAL INSTITUTE FOR THE BLIND (RNIB)

Provides advice and support for people with sight problems

www.rnib.org.uk

DESMOND (Type 2 DIABETES WEBSITE)

Tel: 0116 258 5881

E-mail: desmondweb@uhl-tr.nhs.uk

Website: www.desmond-project.org.uk

NATIONAL SERVICE FRAMEWORK (NSF) FOR DIABETES

This Department of Health document describes the standard of diabetes care you should receive.

www.doh.gov.uk/nsf/iabetes

CARBOHYDRATE EXCHANGE WEBSITE

This website shows you the carbohydrate content of any food you want to find out about.

http://www.eatright.org/cps/rde/xchg/ada/hs.xsl/nutrition_13961_ENU_HTML.htm

DIABETIC RETINOPATHY WEBSITE

Provides information about retinopathy prevention, treatment and research.

www.diabeticretinopathy.org.uk

FEET FOR LIFE

The Society of Chiropodists and Podiatrists website to help with all foot problems.

www.feetforlife.org

NHS DIRECT ONLINE

NHS Direct Online provides health advice and information.

www.nhsdirect.nhs.uk

NETDOCTOR.CO.UK

The UK's leading health website written by doctors and health professionals.

www.netdoctor.co.uk/diabetes/index.shtml

BBC HEALTH DIABETES GUIDE

This guide explains diabetes, its symptoms, causes and treatments.

www.bbc.co.uk/health/diabetes

PREGNANCY AND DIABETES

Is a section on the Diabetes UK website providing useful information and advice.

www.diabetes.org.uk/pregnancy

THE DIABETES TRAVEL INFORMATION WEBSITE

Provides information to help you anticipate any diabetes-related issues before your journey.

www.diabetes-travel.co.uk

MEDICALERT

Medic Alert is a charity providing inscribed jewellery with alerts to health conditions and allergies.

www.medicalert.co.uk

DIABETES INSIGHT

Diabetes Insight provides information and a discussion forum about the condition.

www.diabetes-insight.info

JUEVENILE DIABETES RESEARCH FOUNDATION (JDRF)

JDRF supports Type 1 diabetes in children and young adults

www.jdrf.org

CHILDREN WITH DIABETES

Gives advice about meal planning and nutrition, as well as recipes.

www.childrenwithdiabetes.com

DIABETES RESEARCH & WELLNESS FOUNDATION (DRWF)

The DRWF is an organisation aiming to help people with diabetes to live a healthy life.

www.diabeteswellnessnet.org.uk

THE NATIONAL INSTITUTE FOR HEALTH AND CLINICAL EXCELLENCE (NICE)

NICE is part of the NHS, providing guidance on medications and best practice.

www.NICE.org.uk

The information is also available in Welsh and in large print for the visually impaired.

THE INSULIN PUMP THERAPY GROUP (INPUT)

Helps people access technology to improve their BG control.

Tel: 0800 228 9977

E-mail: info@inputdiabetes.org.uk

Website: www.inputdiabetes.org.uk

MIND

MIND is a charity supporting people with mental health issues.

www.mind.com

GOODMENTALHEALTHMATTERS.COM

Goodmentalhealthmatters.com provides support and information for emotional, psychological and social wellbeing.

goodmentalhealthmatters.com

DIABETIC EXERCISE AND SPORTS ASSOCIATION

A website where you can find out the right kind of exercise for you.

www.diabetes-exercise.org

DISABILITY RIGHTS COMMISSION

Website: www.drc-gb.org

E-mail enquiries: ddahelp@stra.sitel.co.uk

THE ASIAN COOKERY CLUB

Provides information about nutrition and recipes

www.lutonpct.nhs.uk/cookclub.htm

Notes

Further reading

Quick and Easy Cooking for Diabetes

by Jenny Bryan

published by Hodder Wayland

Real Food for Diabetics

by Molly Perham

published by Foulsham

Diabetes Diet Book: Type 2

by Calvin Ezrin

published by Contemporary Books Inc.

Prevent & Cure Diabetes: Delicious Diets, Not Dangerous Drugs

by Sarah Mayhill & Craig Robinson

published by Hammersmith Health Books

Sugarless, Not Flavourless: Delicious Sugar-Free Sweets & Treats That Taste Like the Real Thing

by Catherine Singh

published by CreateSpace Independent Publishing

Family Nutrition Workbook

by Patrick Holford

published by Thorsons, this is a large-print book

Say No to Diabetes

by Patrick Holford

published by Piatkus

The 8-Week Blood Sugar Diet Recipe Book: 150 Simple, Delicious Recipes to Keep Your Blood Sugar Levels in Check
by Claire Bailey & Sarah Schenker
published by Short Books

Nutritional Medicine
by Dr Stephen Davies & Dr Alan Stewart
published by Pan Books

The Better Pregnancy Diet
by Patrick and Liz Holford
 published by ION Press

How to Boost Your Immune System
by Christopher Scarfe
published by ION Press

The GI Diet Pocket Guide
by Rick Gallop
published by Virgin Books

Also by Dr Val Wilson:

Diabetes: The Psychology of Control
Published by Teneo Press

Insulin: Uses and Abuses
Published by Teneo Press

Diabetes: From the Ebers Papyrus to Stem Cell Technology
Published by Teneo Press

GLOSSARY OF TERMS

Acanthosis nigricans – a condition associated with Type 2 diabetes where velvety area of skin develop with increased pigmentation on the back of the neck and armpits. It shows a strong racial disposition and is common in Indian, Hispanic and black populations.

Addison's disease – a condition that affects the adrenal glands that sit on top of the kidneys. The condition can cause frequent and severe hypoglycaemia (low BG levels) because it affects hormones that maintain the amount of glucose in the blood.

Adrenaline – released by the adrenal glands in response to stress, increasing the rate of breathing, heart rate, and improving muscle performance in the fight or flight response.

Alpha-blockers – medications such as Doxazpsin derivatives, used to treat high blood pressure.

Alpha Glucosidase Inhibitors – a group of glucose-reducing medications for the treatment of Type 2 diabetes including Acarbose (Precose) and Miglitadol (Glyset).

Anaemia – iron deficiency.

Anorexia – a disorder where there is an obsessive fear of gaining weight, resulting in severe dietary restriction.

Asthma – a condition characterised by breathlessness due to generalised narrowing of the airways throughout the lungs. There are two different types of asthma in terms of the cause: extrinisic, where external factors (allergens) such as smoke, pollen, dust etc. trigger an attack, and intrinsic, where there is no apparent external cause.

Auto-immune attack – the body's defence mechanism. Type 1 diabetes is an auto-immune disease where the body attacks its own insulin-producing cells in the pancreas.

Auto-immune conditions – conditions caused by auto-immune attack, such as asthma, Type 1 diabetes; coeliac disease and psoriasis.

Auto-immune syndrome – a condition resulting in a high concentration of insulin in the blood despite low blood glucose levels.

Autonomic neuropathy – damage to the autonomic nerves controlling involuntary functions such as digestion and cardiac functions.

Basal rate – the rate of background insulin delivered by an insulin pump that a person needs to keep their BG levels within normal limits without eating or going too high or low.

Bendrofluozide – medication that reduces blood pressure but can increase BG levels.

Beta-carotene – the vegetable form of vitamin A.

Biguanides – a group of glucose-reducing medications for the treatment of Type 2 diabetes including Metformin (Glucophage); Metformin liquid (Riomet); Metformin extended release (Glucophage XR); Foramet (Glumetza).

Bile Acid Sequestrants – a group of glucose-reducing medications for the treatment of Type 2 diabetes including Colesevelam (Welchol).

Blood glucose level – the amount of glucose present in the blood. This varies according to the site where it is measured – blood from the fingertips gives the most up-to-date reading.

Blood plasma – the liquid part of the blood.

BMI – Body Mass Index: 20–20.9 = normal; 25–29.9 = overweight; 30 and above = obese.

Bolus – a dosage of insulin for meals or high BG levels.

Brittle diabetes – Type 1 diabetes that is very difficult to control, with erratic swings in BG from high to low.

Bulimia – a disorder characterised by binge eating, then vomiting and/or laxative abuse.

Calorie – a unit of heat energy (the energy needed to raise the temperature of one kilogram of water by one degree centigrade).

Cannula – a small plastic tube that is inserted under the skin to deliver insulin in insulin pump therapy treatment.

Cataract – a chronic complication of diabetes manifesting as clouding of the lenses of the eyes, impairing vision.

Cardiac arrhythmia – an alteration in the normal heart rhythm.

Cardiomyopathy – a serious condition of the heart and circulatory system thought to stem from damage to the nerves controlling parts of the body not under conscious control, for example, the heartbeat.

Carpal Tunnel Syndrome – a chronic complication of diabetes where the tendons of the hand tighten and draw the fingers into a claw-like position.

CCG – County Commissioning Group, the local Health Authority in every county in the UK who decides on and pays for the funding of treatments such as insulin pump therapy and Continuous Glucose Monitoring to treat Type 1 diabetes.

CDNS – Children's Diabetes Nurse Specialist.

CGM (Continuous Glucose Monitoring) – A piece of technology for use with insulin pump therapy when a plasma glucose sensor is inserted under the skin every 6 days and this is connected to a small transmitter that relays the glucose information to the pump for display to the user to monitor high and low BG levels and act accordingly.

Charcot joints (also known as neuroarthropathy) – a chronic complication of diabetes which refers to the degeneration of, for example, the joints of the foot due to nerve damage, loss of sensation, and areas of pressure.

Cholesterol – blood fats.

Cimetidine – a medication prescribed for indigestion.

Coeliac disease – a systemic condition (having an effect on the whole body) that does not just affect the digestive tract. It is a chronic auto-immune condition triggered by an intolerance to gluten (a protein found in cereal grains such as wheat that is added to bread to make it rise).

Combination Pills – a group of glucose-reducing medications for the treatment of Type 2 diabetes including Pioglitazone & Metformin; Actoplus Met; Glyburide & Metformin (Glucovance); Glipizide & Metformin (Metaglip); Sitagliptin & Metformin (Janumet); Saxagliptin & Metformin (Kombiglyze); Repaglinide & Metformin (Prandimet); Pioglitazone & Glimerpiride (Duetact).

Complications (acute) – hypoglycaemia and diabetic ketoacidosis (DKA) are classed as acute complications of diabetes because they are short-term and can be reversed quickly.

Complications (chronic) – chronic complications of diabetes appear over many years due to high blood glucose levels and can affects any part of the body. The main chronic complications are diabetic retinopathy (affecting the eyes); diabetic neuropathy (affecting the nerves); nephropathy (affecting the kidneys); coronary heart disease; and stroke (affecting the brain).

Condition specific – the knowledge and understanding your partner has about your diabetes and how it affects you.

Corticosteroids – medications that come as tablets, inhalers, injections, or creams used to reduce inflammation.

Cortisol – a hormone released by the adrenal glands when we are stressed which raises blood glucose levels, supresses the immune system and slows digestion.

DAFNE – Dosage Adjustment For Normal Eating – a diabetes education course for people with Type 1.

Depression – the symptoms of depression must be categorised as distressing to the individual, or must cause a decline in social, occupational or other key functions to constitute a diagnosis of depression; symptoms that result from taking illicit drugs or prescription medication, or that arise from bereavement are not counted. Unfortunately, symptoms arising from the burden of self-care for diabetes are also not recognised in making a diagnosis of depression, meaning that the mental and physical toll diabetes takes on the individual is discounted.

DESMOND – Diabetes Education and Self-Management for Ongoing and Newly-Diagnosed – a diabetes education course for people with Type 2 diabetes.

Diabetes insipidus – a rare condition affecting the pituitary gland which manifests as severe thirst and excessive urination that does not contain glucose.

Diabulimia – deliberately omitting or under-dosing on insulin to induce diabetic ketoacidosis and quick weight loss.

Distal polyneuropathy – damage to many of the nerves in the hands and feet.

Diuretics – water tablets that make you urinate more often.

DKA (see ketoacidosis) – the breakdown of fats and protein as an alternative source of energy to glucose which can't be used when there's a lack of insulin, resulting in acid by-products which, in large quantities, cause a medical emergency.

DPP-4 Inhibitors – a group of glucose-reducing medications for the treatment of Type 2 diabetes including Sitagiptin (Januvia); Saxaguptin (Oxglyza) and Linaglyptin (Tradienta).

Dupuytren's disease – refers to a chronic complication seen in people with and without diabetes where the tendons of the wrists and hands tighten and the skin on the palms thickens.

DVLA – Driver and Vehicle Licensing Authority.

eAG – equivalent to HbA1c measurement in the USA.

Electrolytes – minerals like sodium and potassium, needed for nerve and muscle function and to help convert substances like protein into new cells.

Endorphins – hormones that make you feel happy.

Epinephrine (also known as adrenalin) – a hormone that is also used as a medication.

Erectile dysfunction – inability to have or sustain an erection.

Exudates – a mass of cells and fluid that has seeped out of blood vessels or an organ, especially when there is inflammation.

Fair BG control – 7–8 mmol/L

Fasting hypoglycaemia – a condition where blood glucose levels are low due to inadequate stores of glycogen (such as when dieting), or due to the slow conversion of glycogen into glucose when needed. The condition may also be brought about by the consumption of alcohol, and by breast and adrenal cancer.

Fibric acid derivatives – medications used to treat fat disorders.

Fight or flight response – a physical reaction to a perceived harmful event, attack or threat to survival where the options are to fight the threat, run from the threat, or freeze in the hope that the threat won't harm us or because we are paralysed with fear.

Folic acid – vitamin B9.

Foot ulcers – a situation where areas of pressure on the feet cannot be detected as pain and an area of hard skin develops. Over time this continued pressure on this hardened skin causes it to break down and soften until it becomes mushy and comes away, leaving a deep hole, or ulcer, in the foot that becomes infected. If professional help is not sought for a diabetic foot ulcer, the hole becomes larger and the blood supply dies off. At this stage the only thing that can be done is to amputate (possibly the whole of the lower leg) to save the person's life

Gastroparesis – delayed stomach emptying caused by damage to the autonomic nerves.

Gabapentin (also known as Neurontin) – a medication that reduces nerve pain in neuropathy.

Gestational diabetes – develops in 2-4% of women at around 28 weeks of pregnancy.

Gingko biloba – a tree bark traditionally eaten in China to improve blood flow to the arms, legs, fingers and toes. It is still used today and is also thought to improve memory.

Glaucoma – a condition where there is increased pressure within the eyeball, causing gradual loss of sight.

Glucagen hypo kit – a hormone injection that increases BG by slowing down involuntary muscle movement of the stomach and intestines. It is used to treat severe hypoglycaemia when the person is unconscious.

Glucose – a type of sugar formed from the breakdown of glucose.

Glucose intolerance – a term for conditions that increase BG causing hyperglycaemia.

Glucose tolerance factor – a compound containing chromium that helps insulin to regulate BG levels.

Glucose tolerance test – when 75 grams of glucose is given by mouth, a BG result after two hours that is above 7.8 mmol/L (140.4 mg/dl American measurement) but below 11.1 mmol/L (199.8 mg/dl) is generally accepted as impaired glucose tolerance.

Glycaemic Index – the degree to which carbohydrates and starches raise BG relating to the speed that they are absorbed by the body.

Glycogen – glucose (stored carbohydrate) in the liver and body tissues.

Glycogen Storage Disease – a condition where the enzyme which breaks down stored glycogen into glucose is faulty, causing slow-release of glucose by the liver, resulting in hypoglycaemia.

Grave's disease – an enlarged and over-active thyroid gland.

Hashimoto's thyroiditis – a condition causing the thyroid gland to produce less thyroid hormone.

HbA1c (also known as haemoglobin A1c and glycosylated haemoglobin) – measures the amount of glucose that sticks to the red blood cells over a three-month period before they are replaced.

Hereditary Fructose Disorder – a condition causing hypoglycaemia in children because the body can't metabolise (use) natural fruit sugars.

Honeymoon period – can occur in children with Type 1 diabetes where the body's attack on the insulin-producing cells of the pancreas is not sufficient to wipe out all cells as soon as they are formed. When the honeymoon period ends and the pancreas stops producing insulin again in Type 1 diabetes (up to a period of 3 years), BG will begin to rise again.

Hydrocortisone – substances that reduce inflammation.

Hyperglycaemia – high blood glucose levels caused by a lack of insulin.

Hypervitaminosis – a build-up of fat-soluble vitamins A, E, and K in the body.

Hyperstosis – is a condition seen in people with Type 2 diabetes where the vertebrae of the spine fuse together.

Hypoglycaemia – low BG caused by too much insulin, or strenuous exercise, or a lack of food, or because 00has reduced BG.

Hypoglycaemic unawareness – Loss of awareness of the symptoms of low BG, such as tingling or sweating, over time or due to autonomic nerve damage.

Hypostop – glucose gel, treatment for hypoglycaemia.

Hypothermia – a reduction in core body temperature to below 35 degrees centigrade.

Hypothyroidism – an under-active thyroid gland.

Impaired glucose tolerance – where the body is unable to deal with glucose because the action of insulin to bring down BG levels is impaired.

Infusion set – used with insulin pump therapy to deliver insulin via a small cannula placed under the skin and a thin plastic tube going from the cannula to the insulin pump.

Insulin – a hormone produced in the pancreas which controls the amount of sugar (glucose) in the blood.

Insulin insensitivity – the ability of body cells to use insulin correctly to reduce blood glucose levels.

Insulinoma – an insulin-producing tumour, usually benign.

Insulin pump therapy (also known as CSII – Continuous Subcutaneous Insulin Infusion) – a piece of technology that delivers insulin in measured doses directly under the skin.

Insulin Resistance Syndrome – glucose absorption by cells stimulated by insulin is reduced, increasing blood glucose levels and, in response, the amount of insulin that the body produces to cope with these increases.

Intermediate-acting (NPH) insulin – a type of insulin treatment used to treat Type 1 diabetes that covers the BG rise when rapid-acting insulin stops working. It is usually taken twice a day with rapid- or short-acting insulin, taking 1½ to 4 hours to reach the bloodstream where it works for up to 24 hours.

Irritable bowel syndrome (IBS) – a common gut disorder with symptoms such as abdominal pain, bloating, diahorrea and constipation. These symptoms come and go.

Islet cells – the insulin-producing cells of the pancreas.

Ketoacidosis (also known as Diabetic Ketoacidosis or DKA) – the breakdown of fats as an alternative source of energy to glucose which can't be used when there's a lack of insulin, resulting in acid by-products which, in large quantities, cause a medical emergency.

Ketones – products from the breakdown of fats that build up in the blood and are excreted in the urine. Ketone bodies are acids that cause sickness and vomiting when there is high BG.

Kussmaul breathing – rapid breathing or panting that occurs during diabetic ketoacidosis as the body tries to excrete some of the acid build-up via the lungs. The breath smells like acetone (nail polish remover) or pear drops.

LGV – Large Goods Vehicle.

Long-acting insulin – used to reduce BG levels in the treatment of Type 1 diabetes and includes Lantus and Levemir that are usually combined with rapid- or short-acting insulin. It reaches the bloodstream from 40 minutes to 4 hours where it works for up to 24 hours.

Macular degeneration – a condition where the central part of the retina at the back of the eye deteriorates. This is the leading cause of vision loss in people over the age of 60.

Macular oedema – fluid build-up causing loss of vision.

Meglitinides – a group of glucose-reducing medications for the treatment of Type 2 diabetes including Repagunide (Prandin); D-Phenylalanine derivatives; and Nanteglinide (Starlix).

Melatonin – a hormone produced by the pineal gland, the action of which supresses libido in accordance with the fight or flight response by reducing luteinising hormone and follicle stimulating hormone secretion by the anterior pituitary gland.

Metabolic syndrome – a group of associated conditions including coronary heart disease; high blood pressure; high levels of blood fats such as cholesterol; high levels of chemicals that prevent the breakdown of blood clots in the arteries and heart; and obesity.

Metformin – a medication used to treat Type 2 diabetes which lowers BG levels.

Methocloprimide – a medication used for gastroparesis (delayed stomach emptying) that increases muscle contraction in the digestive tract and speeds up the rate of stomach emptying.

Mmol/L – millimoles per litre.

Morbid obesity – a Body Mass Index of 45 and above.

Motor nerve damage – damage to the nerves that carry impulses to the muscles to make them move.

Multiple Daily Injections (MDI) – multiple daily injections or multiple dose insulin.

Necrobiosis lipoidica – a skin condition associated with diabetes where patches of reddish-brown skin form which can become thin and ulcerate.

Neuropathy – the term for nerve damage caused by long-term high BG levels in diabetes.

Nephropathy – a condition caused by hyperglycaemia where the nephrons of the kidney are damaged, impairing function. It is defined as a persistent and clinically detectable level of protein in the urine in association with an elevated blood pressure and reduced kidney function.

Niacin – vitamin B3.

Nocturnal hypoglycaemia – a fall in BG levels when you are asleep.

Normal BG control – 5.0–8.3 mmol/L

Obstructive sleep apnoea – a condition causing intermittent and continual cessation of breathing during sleep, leading to reduced oxygen levels in the blood.

Oedema – fluid that gathers in the lower legs.

Over-active thyroid gland – where the thyroid gland at the front of the neck produces too much thyroid hormone that control metabolism and growth.

Orlistat (Xenical) – a medication that stops around one-third of the fat eaten from being digested.

Ortotist – a specially-trained person at a hospital who makes made-to-measure shoes.

Osteoarthritis – degeneration of the joint cartilage and underlying bone causing pain and stiffness.

Osteopenia – refers to a reduction in bone mass.

Paediatric – relating to children.

PALS – *Patient and Liaison Service.*

Pancreas – a large organ laying behind the stomach that secretes digestive enzymes. Embedded within the pancreas are the Islets of Langerhans which produce insulin.

Pantothenic acid – vitamin B5.

PCV – Passenger Carrying Vehicle.

Peripheral neuropathy – a chronic complication of diabetes which occurs in two forms: diffuse neuropathy, commonly appearing as disorders of sensation in the extremities of the body; and distal polyneuropathy, affecting many nerves of the hands and feet.

Peripheral vascular disease – a circulation disorder that causes blood vessels to become blocked. This can happen in arteries and veins.

Potassium – a mineral that's vital for the healthy function of body cells, tissues and organs and helps control water balance and blood acidity level in the body. It is found in bananas, avocados, spinach, lentils and all fruit and vegetables.

Poor BG control – 9.0 mmol/L and above.

Pre-diabetes (also known as insulin resistance) – is defined as blood glucose concentrations higher than normal, but lower than established limits for diabetes itself.

Prednisone – anti-inflammatory medication.

Primary care – the health care you receive from your General Practitioner (doctor).

Prolactin – a hormone released from the anterior pituitary gland that stimulates milk production after childbirth.

Protein – any of a large group of compounds essential for growth as they are the building blocks of the body.

Psoriasis – an auto-immune condition that affects the skin and joints, causing red, flaky, crusty patches covered with silvery scales appearing on the elbows, knees, scalp and lower back, and joint degeneration. These skin patches can become itchy and sore.

Psychosis – a severe mental disorder where thoughts and emotions are impaired.

Pyridoxine – vitamin B6.

Rapid-acting insulin – a group of insulins taken for the treatment of Type 1 diabetes including Humalog; Novolog and Apidra that is taken before meals to cover the associate BG rise. This is used with long-acting insulin and it takes 10–30 minutes to reach the bloodstream where it works for 3–5 hours.

Reactive hypoglycaemia – low BG levels caused by the pancreas producing too much insulin in reaction, for example, to eating a meal. This DOES NOT happen in people with Type 1 diabetes.

RDA – Recommended Daily Allowance of vitamins and minerals.

Reduced absorption surgery – where the stomach is re-shaped by having around 80% of it removed.

Restrictive surgery – as with reduced absorption surgery to the stomach, restrictive surgery works by physically making the size of the stomach much smaller to slow down digestion to give a feeling of fullness for longer with less food.

Retinopathy – a chronic complication of diabetes which describes a number of symptoms including abnormal dilation of the blood vessels of the eyes; and bleeds in the retina at the back of the eyes. In advanced cases the retina becomes heavily scarred and may lead to blindness.

Retinal photography – screening the eyes for diabetic retinopathy means regular examinations to detect any diabetic changes that could affect sight. These changes are known as *sight-threatening diabetic retinopathy.* Retinal photography will decide whether follow-up treatment from the hospital eye clinic for diabetic retinopathy is needed. If you have no diabetic changes, or if your existing retinopathy is stable, you will be asked to come back for screening a year later.

Retinol – the animal form of vitamin A.

Riboflavin – vitamin B2.

Roaccutane – a synthetic vitamin A supplement called *isotretinoin* that has been associated with birth defects when taken in large dosages of 25,000–500,000 international units per day.

Rosiglitazone – a medication used to lower BG levels in Type 2 diabetes.

Sedentary lifestyle – taking little or no exercise.

Self-efficacy – the self-confidence to do things, like using a BG testing machine, or drawing up and injecting insulin, and building on that to know you can tackle similar challenges.

Sensory nerve damage – diabetic changes to the sensory nerves affecting the ability to feel vibrations, temperature changes and gentle touches to the skin.

Serotonin – a hormone that gives us a sense of wellbeing.

Short-acting insulin – a group of insulins used to treat Type 1 diabetes including Regular (R) insulin taken 30 minutes before a meal to cover the rise in BG. This is used with long-acting insulin and takes 30 minutes to 1 hour to reach the blood stream, and works for 12 hours.

Shoulder adhesive capsulitis – a chronic complication of diabetes describing a condition causing extreme pain and limited movement because the joint capsule has thickened and connective tissue becomes attached to the head of the humerus.

Statins – medication prescribed to lower cholesterol levels.

Stress response – something that makes our palms sweat, gives us heart palpitations, headache, and or diahorrea, tightness in the throat, makes us feel tense, agitated, nauseous, irritated, or short-tempered. Emotionally we feel anxious, uneasy, worried, panic-stricken, angry, or frustrated.

Sugar – a simple carbohydrate that breaks down into glucose in the body.

Sulphonylureas – a group of medications used to reduce BG levels in people with Type 2 diabetes including (Glimepiride (Amaryl); Glyburide (Diabeta, Micronase); Glipizide (Glucotrol, Glucotrol XL); Micronized Glyburide (Glynase); used to lower BG in Type 2 diabetes.

Testosterone – the male sex hormone that stimulates the production of sperm and the development and maintenance of the appearance of male characteristics.

Thiamine – vitamin B1.

Thiazide – diuretic 'water' tablets that make you urinate more which can increase BG levels.

Thiazollidines – a group of BG-lowering medications used to treat Type 2 diabetes including Pioglitazone (TZDS) and Pioglitazone (Actos).

Thrush – a common yeast infection of the vagina that affects most women, especially with diabetes due to raised BG levels. It occurs in warm, moist parts of the body and can also affect the throat (and some men, especially with diabetes).

Transient ischaemia – a partial restriction in blood supply to the brain.

Type 1 diabetes – a condition caused by auto-immune attack on the insulin-producing cells of the pancreas resulting in little or no insulin being available to lower BG levels.

Type 2 diabetes – a condition arising from metabolic syndrome where too much insulin is produced as it is unable to be used by the body to reduce BG levels.

Under-active thyroid gland – a reduction in the amount of thyroid hormone produced by the thyroid gland in the neck.

Unexplained hypoglycaemia – low BG levels that happen for no reason that can't be linked, for example, to exercise, alcohol, drugs, aspirin, or reactive hypoglycaemia.

Visceral fat – fat around the large internal organs of the abdomen.

Vitiligo – a condition where the pigmentation of the skin is lost in Type 1 diabetes as part of the body's autoimmune response to the condition.

Xanthelasma – a skin condition associated with diabetes where small yellow areas (or plaques) appear on the eyelids and other areas of skin which may be an indication of high blood fat (triglyceride) levels.

INDEX

adrenaline (epinephrine)	38, 39, 71, 279
alcohol	40, 64, 73, 113, 128, 219, 285
and blood glucose (BG)	73
carbohydrate content	73
amputation	105, 139, 143, 151, 154
anorexia	188, 279
aspirin	27, 74, 146, 156, 194, 294
protective dose of	74
annual health check	7, 194
asthma inhalers	167
auto-immune destruction	2, 5, 14, 19, 148, 158–159, 279, 280, 282, 291
autonomic neuropathy	45, 139, 140, 144, 145, 280
babies and small children with diabetes	200–203
and blood glucose control	201
and blood glucose monitoring	201
and diabetic ketoacidosis	202
and hypoglycaemia	201–202
and sibling jealousy	202
and Type 2 diabetes	202–203
giving insulin to	201
honeymoon period	201, 286
Bendrofluozide (blood pressure medication)	15, 280
blood glucose (BG)	
alternative site testing	83
how often to test	60, 80
monitoring tests	62,196
Body Mass (BMI)	16–17, 177, 182, 185, 280

brain damage	21, 22, 79
brittle diabetes	22, 121, 280
bulimia	188, 280
cataracts	101, 103, 132, 134, 224
carbohydrates	12, 29, 72, 79, 85–86, 88, 89,93, 110, 162, 174, 209, 226, 285
children's needs	210, 226
content of foods website	90
daily carbohydrate needs	90
cardiovascular function test	194
carers and partners	192, 226, 229– 229
carpal tunnel syndrome	147, 281
Charcot joints	142, 281
cholesterol	7, 70, 87, 91, 97, 127, 132, 139, 145, 146, 155, 176, 194, 281, 288, 293
complaints about diabetes care	189, 198–199
complications	
autonomic nerve disease	45, 139, 140, 144, 145, 280
carpal tunnel syndrome	147, 281
causes	7, 43, 44, 54, 131–134, 149, 151, 176, 182, 282
cataracts	101, 103, 132, 134, 224
Charcot joints	142, 281
Duputren's disease	147, 284
exercising & foot problems	152–153
foot care	143, 152–154, 196, 269
foot ulcers	139, 142, 152, 284
nephropathy (kidney disease)	44, 45, 134, 282, 289

neuropathy (nerve disease)	25, 44, 45, 102, 139–141, 148, 181, 223, 282, 283, 289, 290
of the skin	14, 140, 142, 145, 148, 152, 158
of the spine	287
prevention of	24, 150-153
retinopathy (eye disease)	41, 45, 110, 133–139, 269, 282, 293
shoulder adhesive capsulitis	147, 293
Continuous Glucose Monitoring (CGM)	78, 122, 281
coping strategies	31, 41, 46, 171
DAFNE (Type 1 diabetes education)	21, 160–163, 268, 282
depression	22, 28, 30– 31, 53–57 101–102, 114, 149–150, 176, 184–186, 283
and chemical imbalance	57
and complications	30. 53, 55, 149
and emotions	56, 170
helping yourself	44, 55–57
symptoms of	53–54, 150–151, 186, 223, 283
treatment	57, 150
DESMOND (Type 2 diabetes education)	29, 165–171, 173, 269, 283
diabetes insipidus	5, 283
diabetic foods	211
diabetic ketoacidosis (DKA)	63–65, 73, 213, 214, 282, 283
causes	64, 213–214, 283
diabulimia	65, 212, 213, 283
ketones	63, 65, 66, 71, 110, 192, 198, 213, 288

Kussmaul breathing	64, 288
symptoms	64
treatment	65–66
diabetic nephropathy	44, 45, 134, 282, 289
diabetic neuropathy	25, 44, 45, 102, 139–141, 148, 181, 223, 282, 283, 289, 290
diabetic retinopathy	41, 45, 110, 133–139, 269, 282, 293
diabulimia	65, 212, 213, 283
diagnosis	
and ethnicity	15
and drugs	15
and genetics	14–15
and illness	14, 15
driving and hypos	16
informing the DVLA	25
Duputren's disease	147, 283
eAG	22, 283
elderly	
and diet	222–223, 225
and eyesight	223, 224
and exercise	223
and symptoms of diabetes	221, 222
care homes and diabetes	225, 226
choosing their own care	222, 226
elderly-onset Type 2	220, 221
Help The Aged charity	223
medication	225
mental functioning and diabetes	222, 225
preventing complication in	24
urinary and sexual problems	221, 224
emotions	
anger	28, 33–36, 51, 53, 56
anxiety	32–33, 101, 102, 114, 183, 185, 188, 202
blaming yourself	31–32
denial	28–31, 48, 53
fear	42–45, 55, 218, 220

guilt, dealing with		37–38
relief		47–48
exercise		
	and burning calories	84, 167
	and complex carbohydrates	72
	and hypoglycaemia	24, 68
	and hyperglycaemia	61. 71, 72
	and complications	153. 223
	intense	24, 71, 72
	moderate	24, 68, 69
	with foot problems	152–153
eye screening (for retinopathy)		134–139
famous diabetic		30
fasting hypoglycaemia		73, 203, 284
fat		8, 13, 16, 17–18, 69, 112, 113, 145, 149, 156, 187
	low-fat foods	85, 174, 211
fear		42–45, 55, 218, 220
	of change	42–46
	of complications	43–44
	of needles	42–43
	of night-time hypoglycaemia	76, 218
	of pain	44–45
	of the reaction of others	45, 51, 57, 124, 172
	overcoming	43–44, 46–47
fight or flight response		38, 279, 284, 288
food choices		161, 164, 165, 169, 195, 210, 211
food labels		85, 90, 92, 202
fruit and veg		92, 93, 167
	portion size	93
further reading		276–278
	also by Val Wilson	278

Gabapentin 45, 141, 285

gestational diabetes 5, 18, 109, 111, 285

glaucoma 133, 224, 285

glucose

    glucose-lowering tablets 4, 12, 62, 124–127, 225

glucagen injection kit 22, 67, 76, 79, 80, 202, 208, 218, 285

glycaemic index 86, 285

glycogen 13, 14, 159, 284, 285

gingko biloba 27, 285

going into hospital 189, 196, 198

good blood glucose control 7, 22, 121, 201, 219

HbA1c

    and pregnancy 61, 62. 110. 113, 123, 177

    table % to mmol/L 62

HbA1c test 22, 23, 24, 44, 60, 61, 62, 71, 82, 109, 151, 174, 179, 204, 215, 223, 286

healthy eating 19, 173

high blood pressure 70, 98, 102. 103, 110, 132,133, 144, 145, 146, 155, 156, 176, 188, 194, 279, 288

high-sugar foods 86, 87

how many people have diabetes? 6–7

How many have undiagnosed diabetes? 8–9

hypoglycaemia

    causes 62, 66–80

    exercise and 24, 71

    fasting hypoglycaemia

Glucagen injection kit 22, 67, 76, 79, 80, 202, 208, 218, 285

    how severe hypo feels 79–80

hypo-busting tips 209–210
hypoglycaemia unawareness 26, 121
mild 21, 74, 75, 112
night-time hypos 76, 77, 289
severe 22, 67, 75–76,
79, 159, 285

sulfonylureas and 68, 74, 82, 125, 197
symptoms of 75–76

hyperglycaemia 29, 49, 63, 71, 72,
81, 111, 213, 285

insulin
and heat 46
injection and pens 116
injection sites 119
insulin inhalers 119

insulin pump therapy 43, 78, 120–124, 143,
144, 204, 207, 271, 281

intermediate-acting 117
in Type 2 diabetes 23
long-acting 117
multiple daily injections 43, 121, 204, 289
rapid-acting 116
short-acting 116
storage and use 118

insulin pump therapy 43, 78, 120–124, 143,
144, 204, 207, 271, 281

insulin resistance 17, 70, 91, 129, 145,
158, 176, 188, 202,
212, 216, 287, 290

islet cells 20, 287, 290
joint and muscle pain 146
lifestyle change 72, 124, 173, 174, 176,
185

low-sugar foods 86, 92

macular degeneration   133, 284, 288
medications that increase blood glucose
     blood pressure tablets   15, 77, 156, 280
     corticosteroids   64, 156, 282
     statins   155, 293
     thiazide (water tablets   155, 293
     vitamin B3 (nicotinic acid)   155, 293
     Prednisone   15, 290

psychosis medications   156

medications that reduce blood glucose
     antibiotics   156
     alpha-blockers   156
     aspirin   27, 74, 146, 156, 194, 294

     corticosteroids   64, 156, 282
     fibric acid medication   156, 284
     fish oil supplements   156
     heroin   156
     sleeping pills   156
     water tablets (diuretics)   64, 155, 156, 283

medical conditions that increase blood glucose
     coeliac disease   14, 95, 157, 279, 282
     psoriasis   14, 158, 279, 291
     thyroid disorders   14, 98, 127, 157, 158, 285, 286, 289, 294

medical conditions that reduce blood glucose
     Addison's disease   158, 279
     auto-immune syndrome   159, 280
     glycogen storage disorder   159, 285
     hereditary fructose disorder   159, 286
     insulinoma   159, 287
     malaria   159
     pneumonia   159
     severe lack of oxygen   159

Memantine medication   45, 141
metabolic syndrome   183, 288, 294

minerals	95–100, 102–103
arrhythmia (cardiac)	96, 281
deficiency symptoms	95–100
electrolytes	95, 284
ketoacidosis (DKA)	63–65, 73, 213, 214, 282, 283
sources and purpose	95–98
moods	
and blood glucose	48–52, 170–171
and mental health	51, 54, 183, 185, 188, 189, 273
and self-care	55, 149
and understanding of others	49, 51–52
Multiple Daily Injects (MDI)	43, 121, 204, 289
myths about diabetes	19–27
neuropathy (nerve damage)	25, 44, 45, 102, 139–141, 148, 181, 223, 282, 283, 289, 290
treatments for	44–45, 285
nephropathy (kidney disease)	44, 45, 134, 282, 289
normal blood glucose control	2, 22, 55
obstructive sleep apnoea	187, 289
pancreas	2, 5, 13, 14, 19, 20, 37, 113, 149, 155, 159, 167, 201, 279, 286, 287, 290, 294
perfect control	22–23
pre-diabetes	145. 290
Primary Care	7, 291
pregnancy	
and complications	110, 112
and gestational diabetes	5, 18, 109, 111, 285
and large babies in diabetes	112, 113
quality of life	72, 176, 185

recipes	232–267
relationships	58–59, 142, 227–229
retinopathy (eye disease)	41, 45, 110, 133–139, 269, 282, 293
reversing Type 2 diabetes	
and low-carbohydrate diets	174–175
and low-fat diets	173–174
and quality of life	72, 176, 185
stigma of having Type 2	172, 184
with weight-loss surgery	178–179
school-age children with diabetes	
and Children's Diabetes Nurse	206
and continuous glucose sensor	78, 122, 281
and DAFNE	210
and dietary needs	210–211
and exercise	207, 210
and glucagen hypo injection kit	208
and hypoglycaemia	202, 207, 209
and insulin pump therapy	205, 207
and ketone testing	208
and multiple daily injections	204, 206
diabetic foods	211
hypo-busting tips	209–210
sedentary lifestyle	17, 292
self-efficacy (self-confidence)	51, 292
sex	101, 108, 113–115
erectile dysfunction	113–115, 144, 224, 284
reduced sex drive in women	108
sharing diabetes care	190. 192, 195, 198, 228, 230
shoulder adhesive capsulitis	147, 293
skin	14, 140, 142, 145, 148, 152, 158
sleep	
and insulin	187, 289
and obstructive sleep apnoea	187, 289
effects of shift work	187, 289
slow wound healing	101, 141
smoking	31, 37, 40, 84, 105,

	106, 154,
and amputation	106, 154
benefits of stopping	106
and diabetes	65, 106, 154
statins	155, 293
starches and sugars	85–90, 285
stress	20, 25, 28, 35, 38–42,
	53, 293
dealing with	40–42
effect on diabetes	38–40
symptoms	38–39
stress response	293
students away from home	215–220
and adverse coping strategies	217–218
and hypoglycaemia	217–218
and social activities	216–217
and support for managing diabetes	219–220
stroke	74, 105, 106,
	146, 155, 282
sweet things	21
teenagers with diabetes	
and changing to adult diabetes clinic	212
and diabetic complications	211, 212
and diabetic ketoacidosis risk	211
and hormonal changes	214
and independence	211
and peer pressure	211
and resisting authority	211
and weight issues	211
diabulimia	65, 212–213, 283
text reminders from the hospital	214–215
thiazide (diuretics/water tablets)	155, 293
Type 1 diabetes	
causes	2, 5
symptoms	4, 11, 12
diagnosis	14, 15

Type 2 diabetes 4, 5, 6
 causes 3, 4, 8, 11, 12
 symptoms 4, 15, 16–19
 in children 5, 6, 188, 202–203
 risks 5, 7, 16, 18, 19, 70, 72, 84, 145, 176, 179

useful contacts 268–272

vascular disease 114, 145–146, 290
vertebra (spine) 287

vitamins
 deficiency 100–103
 fat-soluble 94–95
 needs in diabetes 92, 154
 Orlistat, effects of 95
 RDA 99–100, 191
 sources and purpose 93–94
 water-soluble 95

waist measurement 17
 and visceral fat 18, 294

weight
 calorie needs 104
 low-carbohydrate diets 174, 175
 low-fat diets 173–174

weight-loss surgery
 and excess skin 186, 187
 and lifestyle change 177
 and self-confidence 187
 and vitamin deficiency 178
 complications of surgery 180–181
 counselling and support 186–187
 effects of surgery on diabetes 176, 178, 179
 eligibility for 185
 expectations of 186
 for overweight children 183
 how much weight is lost? 183–184

psychological consequences of	183–184
your diabetes care team	190–191
your responsibilities	195–196
your rights	
and general heal care	189–190
and specific diabetes care	190–195
complaints	189, 198–199

Printed in Great Britain
by Amazon